THE ART OF MIDLIFE

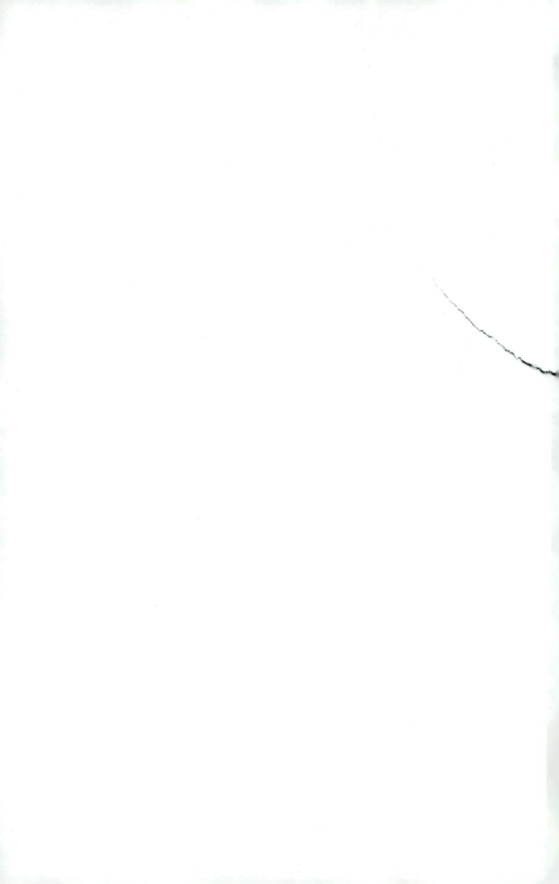

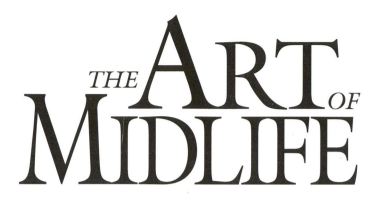

THE ART OF MIDLIFE

COURAGE AND
CREATIVE LIVING
FOR WOMEN

LINDA N. EDELSTEIN

BERGIN & GARVEY
Westport, Connecticut • London

Library of Congress Cataloging-in-Publication Data

Edelstein, Linda N.
    The art of midlife : courage and creative living for women / Linda
N. Edelstein.
      p. cm.
    Includes bibliographical references (p.) and index.
    ISBN 0–89789–580–0 (alk. paper)
    1. Middle aged women—Psychology. 2. Middle aged women—
Attitudes. 3. Aging—Psychological aspects. 4. Self-actualization
(Psychology) I. Title.
HQ1059.4.E34 1999
305.244—dc21   98–20126

British Library Cataloguing in Publication Data is available.

Library of Congress Catalog Card Number: 98–20126
ISBN: 0–89789–580–0

First published in 1999

Bergin & Garvey, 88 Post Road West, Westport, CT 06881
An imprint of Greenwood Publishing Group, Inc.
www.greenwood.com

Printed in the United States of America

The paper used in this book complies with the
Permanent Paper Standard issued by the National
Information Standards Organization (Z39.48–1984).

10 9 8 7 6 5 4 3 2

To my daughters, Keira and Jennifer,
and to all our daughters

❖ ❖ ❖

Contents

Acknowledgments
xi

Introduction
1

PART I: RELINQUISH THE OLD
5

1
"Freedom Is Daily, Prose-Bound, Routine Remembering"
An Overview of Midlife Creativity
7

2
"The Terrible Weight of All This Unused Life"
Relinquish the Old
17

3
"Glowing Coals under Grey Ashes"
Midlife
31

4
"First It Was in Black and White,
and Then It Was in Color"
Creativity and Insight
49

PART II: RECONNECT TO THE SELF
71

5
"She Must Braid Us All Together"
The Psychology of Women
73

6

"I Am Her Only Novel"
Relationships with Parents and Their Dreams for Us
91

7

"There's Still So Much I'd Like to See"
How We Are Formed by Social Forces
99

8

"Once You Are Real You Can't Be Ugly"
Authenticity
111

9

"Finding a Fortune in the Lining of an Old Coat"
Aggression and Creativity
125

10

"The Long Meandering Fingers of Ice Will Thicken"
Problems in Creative Living
143

PART III: REFOCUS THE FUTURE
159

11

"Life Shrinks or Expands in Proportion
to One's Courage"
Finding Courage
163

12

"Don't Dream It, Be It"
Turning Points
171

13

"I Have a Brain and a Uterus and I Use Both"
Women and Work
181

Contents

14
"Let the Beauty You Love Be What You Do"
Achievements and Dreams
191

Epilogue
201

Bibliography
203

Index
211

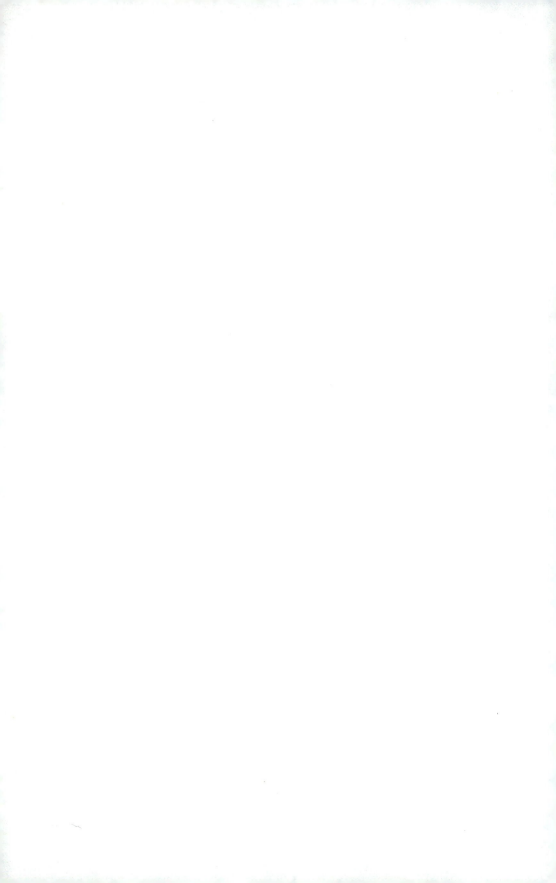

❖ ❖ ❖

ACKNOWLEDGMENTS

I want to acknowledge the generosity of others. Early publishing advice came from Rowena McDade, M.S.W. Suggestions on the proposal came from Kathleen Slomski, M.B.A., and actual editing was done by Lee Rodin, M.S.W., and Fred Shafer, M.A. Good friends and talented colleagues read and critiqued the manuscript in different stages. Gloria Gallo, Ph.D., read the chaotic early draft and gave me the encouragement I badly needed. Very helpful comments came from Ellen Dresner, L.S.W., Hedda Leonard, Anita Adams, M.B.A., and my literary agent, Loretta Weingel-Fidel. Lisa Stolley, M.A., gently edited a later draft of the manuscript. Maria Fay, Peg White, M.L.S., and Steve Schmidt, M.L.S., librarians extraordinare, helped with final drafts. Martha Cristensen worked on the index. Charlie Waehler, Ph.D., also living with a book, and Margit Kir-Stimon, Ph.D., provided warm support and advice at many intervals during this process. Mark Epstein, J.D., Eve Epstein, J.D., and the other members of my second family, Charna, David, and Daniel Epstein, were regularly treated to all my ups and downs and remained remarkably sympathetic throughout. At Greenwood, thanks to Nita Romer, Editor, and Karen D. Treat, Production Supervisor.

I belong to several creative communities. Much of my thinking was confirmed by the women attending the fourth Chicago Professional Women's Conference, "A Weekend's Worth of Creativity," organized by Nancy Newton and myself. The students in "Separation, Loss and Mourning," a course I have taught for years at the Chicago School of Professional Psychology, have always provided inspiration by their interest. The Sunday Writing Group, with Margit, Nancy, and Kathleen, remains a high point of every month.

Finally, I turned the manuscript over to Nancy Newton, Ph.D., who, having already discussed these ideas with me for years, was also pressed into service to edit my words, check my thinking, and smooth out my uneven writing voice, all of which she did with her usual grace. She even read the notes. My most personal sources for confidence and courage remain Jennifer and Keira, my daughters. Thank you. I am blessed to have all these people in my life.

My deep appreciation goes to all the women who allowed me to enter and record a period of their lives. Women I interviewed and all the women I have worked with in therapy made themselves vulnerable in order to continue to go forward. It is always an honor to be invited into someone's life. I am endlessly heartened and amazed at the honesty of women who willingly open their lives because of concern and connection with other women they will never meet.

❖   ❖   ❖

INTRODUCTION

The heart of my work is clinical psychotherapy, and in that practice, I have found a great many unanswered questions. Some resonate strongly with my own. One question—how can we, as midlife women, author intentional, spirited lives?—is the basis for this book. Because of who I am professionally, I turned my interest in midlife creativity into research and went about it in several ways simultaneously.

I reviewed the theories that examined women's adult development, loss and adaptation, and creativity. I located relevant research studies in psychology and distilled hundreds of pages of psychological research and thinking into what I hope is intelligent, conversational language. Theory and research were both necessary because I needed to confirm or refute my ideas and I wanted to integrate three processes that are usually treated as distinct: mourning, creativity, and normal developmental change. In addition, I looked for, found, interviewed, transcribed, and analyzed talks with women who had refashioned themselves in satisfying ways and had carried out interesting and significant changes in their lives. I interviewed women—*ordinary women*, not the rich and famous—in the Midwest, where I live, and elsewhere. The women, who ranged in age from their late thirties to their late fifties, told me about all kinds of changes—leaving jobs, starting businesses, returning to artistic pursuits, marriages, searches for biological parents, and unfortunate events such as deaths, divorces, handicaps, or alcoholism—that became sources of motivation to build new lives. Essential to this project was the fact that the women experienced the changes as being within their power, a happy contrast to the adaptation research I had done years ago with women whose children had died unexpectedly. Those deaths were tragedies that entered women's lives like bricks through glass and shattered them just as easily. From those women, I learned about overwhelming losses and limitless mourning. For this book, I sought women who had choices about the changes in their lives and made decisions that led to positive outcomes. What does it take to create a full second half of life?

The twenty interviews provide the major descriptions and illustrations, but I have used other information as well, all disguised. During the last fifteen years, I have probably worked with more than one hundred clients in their middle years. With permission, some small portions of their stories are included. A few examples are composites of the experiences of several women. True stories also come from autobiographies and biographies. I recount some of my own insights, which were the most difficult to put honestly on paper. The final source is literature; I found a few fictional characters who were too good to pass up.

The women who speak throughout the chapters will provide you with a sense of community. I believe they will inspire you as they have inspired me, and give you courage and direction as well. It helps us to see the efforts of other women because through their experiences we recognize our own experiences as valid and are guided by their labors. The women I spoke with had at times felt lost, stale, and unhappy, but they were not disturbed women—they were well-functioning, high-achieving, articulate, and creative women who were willing to take emotional risks. Each told of reaching a moment when she heard her own buried voice, found courage, and responded.

I came to think about midlife creativity as a process of three general steps. Therefore, the book is organized into three sections that follow the unfolding process—relinquishing, reconnecting, and refocusing. Chapters in Part I explain how women relinquish the old ways: the losses we grieve, the necessity of mourning in middle age, the opportunities presented to us, and how we can approach the process with creativity and insight. The chapters in Part II discuss the challenges of reconnection to ourselves. First, we look at reconnection as it applies to the psychological forces that shape women's experiences: separation and connection, relationships with parents and their dreams for us, and the social forces that had such enormous impact on the baby boomer generation. Second, we examine reconnection through the issues women face in midlife: authenticity, confidence, entitlement, acceptance, and anger. In the final chapter of this section, I describe problems and obstacles to creative growth. We look at these problems to solve them, not to get stuck in them. Part III is devoted to refocusing our futures, and includes chapters on work, new definitions of courage, actual turning points, and achievements.

A disclaimer! In this book, I point out that we have often been sold the *truth* of what is *good* for us as women and what is *right* for us as women. Assumptions based on men's lives have been applied to women's experiences. These conjectures have covered women like suffocating blankets, and in the process, driven us further from understanding ourselves. I do not want to duplicate the behaviors that I criticize. We do not all remember the same things, respond in the same ways, or care to the same degree. Different forces impact each individual, and our innate personalities always play a major part in our reactions. Also, there is profound diversity within generations and among those of different sexual orientations, races, ethnic backgrounds, educational levels, political leanings, and more. Furthermore, many ideas in this book are not exclusive to women, midlifers, or baby boomers; many events affect all generations, not just ours; and many experiences are universal. I also know that there are profound similarities between women and men, but men have been studied since psychology began, and as women, we need some time to tell our stories. I am not presenting your truth. I am presenting, however, hard-won, interesting ideas from which you can build your truth. In spite of the multitude of individual differences that exist, I believe that significant, common experiences have shaped our lives as women. I am sufficiently convinced to write these ideas down on paper and let others use them, reshape them, and work toward increased understanding. I have never liked self-help books because they make change seem quick and easy, and that has certainly not been true for me. Change takes work, and these chapters make it increasingly clear why change is a difficult but vital and rewarding aspect of life.

In reading this book, you may feel, as did the women I interviewed and as did I when I was writing, a mixture of emotions—angry and sad that learning takes so long, touched by the simple moments that capture a rare honesty, and excited by discovery. I wanted this book to be accessible, reader friendly. I wanted it to be the kind of book that I enjoy reading; maybe my daughters would read it. The stories are moving because the women were honest in telling them. After reading autobiographies, but even more so after each interview, I was elated to belong to this generation of women. I hope that I have transmitted some of the inspiration I received.

I would like very much to hear about your experiences at midlife. If you would like to describe your midlife changes, please e-mail me at Midlifeart@aol.com.

❖ ❖ ❖

PART I
RELINQUISH THE OLD

❖ 1 ❖

"FREEDOM IS DAILY, PROSE-BOUND, ROUTINE REMEMBERING"
An Overview of Midlife Creativity

What I wanted was to be myself again.
 —Sandra Hochman

So in the long run, it didn't matter if you had been good or not. The girls in high school who had "gone all the way" had not wound up living in back alleys in shame and disgrace, like she thought they would; they wound up happily or unhappily married, just like the rest of them.
 —Fannie Flagg

I have been present at many inspiring moments. I have glimpsed change and growth in the women with whom I work, and feel a deep joy at these times. This book tries to capture the experiences of some of the women I have worked with and many others I have met. *The Art of Midlife: Courage and Creative Living for Women* examines the midlife years of ordinary women who imaginatively recreated their lives. I have included psychological understanding of how they did it, how they transformed "I'm getting older and I'm stuck" into "Life is precious and it belongs to *me!*" This transformation is a production in three acts—relinquishing the old, reconnection to the self, and refocusing the future. The steps also refer to the emphasis of our attention—relinquishing refers to our pasts, reconnection looks at our past and present lives, and refocusing accentuates the present and future.

The work of the past is to relinquish youth and all that it means to each of us. At midlife, normal aging requires us to let go, to mourn. Letting go frees us from roles in our lives that have become outdated or ill fitting and liberates energy for a full life in the present.

Reconnecting to ourselves involves understanding the women we are today. We haven't just grown older; we have also grown up. Perhaps our lives now require new directions or simplicity; perhaps we have misplaced some essential element and need to dig it out of the odds and ends we have accumulated.

Refocusing moves us into the future; it involves developing lives that take us forward. The idea of life as an intentional, personal creation becomes a new way to look at daily choices, and midlife is the ideal time to get moving.

Melanie tells her story with a purity that permits us to glimpse all the processes that will be looked at again in the pages to come. I had known Melanie only as a neighbor before we sat down to talk. She was forty-nine, dark and shining, and very Greek, with a simple artistic elegance to her clothes, hair, and jewelry. She spoke with a directness and animation that captured my attention completely. I learned that she was the daughter of Greek immigrants and had worked with her father in the family grocery store from age six. Her father was her "soul mate"; he expected a great deal from her and she would have burst her heart to deliver. When he said, "count the change," Melanie, terrible in math but more fearful of being a disappointment to her proud, beaming father, counted the change. "I could have been four and I would have been a cashier!" she insisted. He died when she was only fifteen. Life changed then; he was gone, and her mother became depressed for several years. It took Melanie's injury in a car accident to shake her mother back into the present.

Melanie had been an artist since childhood and trained as a painter in school, but that life became impossible to continue in young adulthood, with two young daughters to raise alone after her divorce. At forty-nine, she was vice president for development in a large Chicago not-for-profit organization, supervising a staff of twenty-seven, with endless fund raising and social activities to oversee. She had been with Timothy, a successful businessman, for nine years, and was undecided about marriage but not about the permanence of their commitment to each other. They were deeply involved with each other's lives and children, creating a noisy, semiblended family.

After I listened to Melanie, I knew I would write this book. She epitomized all that I knew and hoped about venturing ahead. She laughingly began the interview by saying, "The last thing Tim said to me when I was walking out the door was, 'Don't talk too much.' I said, 'She's not going to use my real name. I'll be Melanie.'"

MELANIE'S STORY

Melanie felt the beginning rumbles of change in her midforties, after her younger daughter left for the West Coast.

Dita was going into her first year of college. I had become completely overwhelmed with my motherhood. I felt that my mothering was insufficient. I was overwhelmed by the most tremendous guilt. So (a) she was going far away, and (b) I was taking stock of my life. I suppose I was also in a low point in my relationship with Tim. . . . I felt like I was doing all the compromising. I was disillusioned and disappointed. I had given this relationship nine years. . . . I was beating myself up something awful.

Melanie went into therapy, and one of the first issues she had to grapple with was her desire to be a superstar in everything, including mothering. Her imperfect caretaking fueled her guilt.

When Dita came back at Thanksgiving I had this ceremony that I called The Ceremony of Roots and Wings. To me it was life or death. . . . I gave [my daughters] little jars filled with things, and I wrote prayers, and we held hands and I lit a candle, and basically I asked them to forgive me and I forgave them. They were sitting here in the living room thinking, "Oh God, Mom has flipped." They didn't understand what was going on, but they felt that it was very important to me and very emotional, and somehow that stuck with them. After it was over, they asked me why I did it. When I was raising them, screaming like a banshee, I was an idiot. I think it was the pressure of raising them and of being so totally responsible for them in this very hostile world and feeling very alone. So I told the kids, "When I'm dead, I don't want you all screwed up because you're feeling guilty for the stupid things we did to each other when you were in high school." And that was really true. So we did that.

By November, I had gotten over Dita going to school, and I started to work on my relationship, that, at the moment, wasn't doing it for me.

Not an unusual story; it belongs to us all—children launched, relationship worries, reaching the middle years. Melanie was relinquishing youth and her role as mom to at-home children, which gave her time to think about herself, her life, her dissatisfactions, and the dynamics of the important relationships in her life, past and present. As we see next, she was going to let go of much more.

She realized that there was a powerful connection between her past need to be a superstar in an effort to please her father and her present need to fulfill overly high expectations for herself as a mother. This insight led Melanie to see that these twin themes, her wish to please others and her automatic inclination to fulfill their expectations, showed up in other areas of life too, particularly in her attitude toward work and her behavior in her present relationship with Tim. She said, "I was living up to [my father's] expectations. . . . That has been the program. That is how I was programmed into jobs. I was programmed with Tim, except none of it was bringing me any happiness. So suddenly . . . I was able to think about myself for the first time since my father died when I was fifteen." Because her father had died unexpectedly when she was young, Melanie had never had the opportunity to separate from him in an age-appropriate way. She carried the excessive desire to be perfect far into adulthood, where, like many women, she was raising children, working, paying the mortgage, and living each day—without much time for herself.

Melanie's first steps toward change were to recognize the outdated ways she behaved and felt. This included her guilt over insufficient mothering and her persistent attempts to meet other people's expectations. The mourning was about letting go of these outdated reactions: being a superstar, being perfect, pleasing difficult people. Melanie called her behavior "programmed" because it started years ago, but her actions continued as automatic responses in relation to other people. Similar behaviors were showing up in disguised forms in the present, and the result was that Melanie felt dissatisfied, unhappy, and lost. As she reconnected with herself, she recognized the formation of her wishes as well as their present futility.

She had to face these and other unpleasant behaviors. Melanie saw that she had used work to fill the empty space in her life. "Now, I had time to think about myself. I hadn't let myself do that too much because I took every available space that was left and filled it with work. . . . I thought the institution drove me, but I realized I drove them." She found emotions and behaviors that needed to be understood. "Somewhere, maybe two years into that four-year period, I guess I started to see myself more for who I was, and it was okay."

Reconnection brought additional insights. The processes of relinquishing the old and reconnecting to herself were not only about letting go. These steps uncovered the confident artist who acquired respect for her own judgments and put her in touch, for the first time, with the wants and needs that she had surrendered years before. There was a moment when all this learning and the emotion came together with force.

I think I was really angry at Tim. I was blaming him; he made mistakes too, but I wasn't forgiving at that point. I was angry. I think that anger was helpful because it precipitated what I think was my watershed experience.

His son was newly married to Lisi, who was this very difficult person, but I was her advocate. I made everyone make nice. I was being really supportive of Lisi. Then she wanted to come to Christmas Eve. I didn't feel comfortable having her at Christmas Eve because that was a very close family thing. I never had company on Christmas Eve, none of my friends, none of Tim's family or friends, none of my best friends, and Tim's family did not celebrate Christmas, so I said that I would rather that she come on Christmas Day. She kept pushing. I started to get vibes that this was . . . "I'm the Queen of the Hop."

Tim's sons and Lisi joined Melanie's family for a lavish dinner on Christmas Day. Tim had given Melanie a video camera the night before, and even though all gifts had been put away, Lisi found the camera and asked to borrow it. Melanie did not respond, not liking to "loan anything to anyone." Lisi later called and asked to borrow the camera and was told, "No, it was too new."

"Tim begged me not to do this, said it would cause trouble; I asked, 'Is the camera mine or the family's? They asked me and I gave them an answer.' Tim railed, but I hung in; it was a catastrophe." Tim's son and daughter-in-law didn't speak to him for five months following this incident, and then, at a family meeting arranged for the purpose of reconciliation, Tim's children surprised him and brought up old childhood issues for the first time, reaching back many years to criticize him for the divorce from their mother. Tim was deeply hurt.

Tim said, "The gun was loaded, but you pulled the trigger," but I said, "No, the elephant is in the living room and it is your elephant, not mine." I drew my line. I hung in there, against all this. It was like the Dr. Seuss story of Yertle the Turtle, the King of the Pond, who climbs up on top of all these turtles so he can see the moon, but there is a little turtle in the middle named Ned who hiccups, and the kingdom comes toppling down. I felt like Ned because suddenly the whole family is around me in ruins, saying that it was Melanie and the video camera. Tim said I was selfish, that I should have understood that it would hurt him and his family and I should not have done this.

The video camera episode was like the tip of an iceberg; it was the only part that showed, although a mountain existed below the surface. For Melanie, reconnecting with herself was no longer about her past, but about her present. She had not reached her forties without learning a lot about people; she was confident in her judgment, and she liked herself. This was a turning point for Melanie in her relationships with people. She was freed from the daily worries about her daughters' welfare, she had gotten tired of being the peacekeeper in Tim's family, and she recognized her overdeveloped instinct to please difficult people. Melanie's reaction to Lisi's demands confirmed, finally, that she was no longer willing to put everyone else's needs before her own.

Peace at any price, something I would have subscribed to before that. . . . Suddenly they couldn't believe that I wasn't capitulating. This little *Leave It to Beaver* story was when I realized that I had the courage and the strength to tell everyone to take one big flying leap. Slowly I built my confidence up. . . . I started drawing my lines more and more, and it really raised havoc. Melanie's drawing a line! What do you mean? Melanie never draws lines! Melanie turns herself into a pretzel! It wasn't like all this was happening and people were saying, "Oh, Melanie drew a line and we are going to be very careful not to step over it." But it didn't make any difference. I drew lines with my children, too. I was more clear about things. I apologized when I made mistakes; I just could discern better what I was doing, and could draw my lines.

Melanie's turning point was one in which she used her own judgment and stuck to it, not out of the rebelliousness or the stubbornness of youth, but because she trusted her judgment. She held the belief that the camera was hers to keep or loan as she saw fit, and pleasing people did not have to be the deciding dynamic. At another time of life, Melanie might not have even perceived the choice, or she might have resolved to sacrifice her wants in favor of family harmony. In those instances, when the children were young or when she was afraid that she would lose Tim's love, she might have come to a different decision from the one she reached at Christmas. Another decision would have been neither good nor bad, simply different. But that year, at forty-seven years old, Melanie made the choice not to share, not to dominate Tim's daughter-in-law, but also not to respond submissively to Lisi's demands. As she so humorously but poignantly described, it was a new behavior to draw lines, not to give in, not to make peace, and the others reacted badly at first, waiting for the old Melanie to give in.

I think I needed one giant event. I think that stupid video camera event turned the corner for me. I did something that nobody wanted me to do. The man I love was blaming me for killing his family. I hung in there. I did it anyway, and when it was all over, everyone agrees and acknowledges that it wasn't the video camera; I was not to blame. There was nothing, nothing wrong with anything that I did. I guess I feel somewhat vindicated. I trusted my judgment better, I trusted myself better, I valued myself more, I respected myself more because I was dealing with losing everything. I was going to lose Tim, his kids, and I didn't care. "I will lose all of you over this if the only way I can have you is to sell my soul to keep the peace. I'm not selling my soul," I said to Timothy. "I am not selling my soul to you, to my kids, to your kids, to anyone. I'm not selling my soul to anyone. I don't care how good it would have been for you or anyone. It was selling my soul." When I really came to grips with selling my soul—when you begin to think like that, you think, "Who are you? What do you stand for?"

The other central midlife issue that was going on for Melanie at this time was her personal confrontation with mortality. At this time, for many women, parents are aging or may have died, we feel our own aging process, illness may strike, or, as in Melanie's case, a friend dies.

One of her dear friends had died, and Melanie had been at her bed during those last weeks. This forced Melanie to confront the finiteness of life in a very personal way. When Lois died, Melanie faced her own dread of being alone, no longer as a fifteen-year-old whose father died, but as an adult woman. In easing the last days for Lois, Melanie's fear of dying dropped away. Facing the finiteness of one's own life can have different results; it could have stopped Melanie cold and led her to settle in, perhaps mildly depressed, and wait twenty or thirty years for her turn, but Lois's death did not do that. Facing the finiteness of life furnished motivation for Melanie to live fully, to cherish life. She gained confidence in her ability to face life, even alone. The result of this experience was that she developed a different view, not of dying, but of living. Her friend's death gave her courage.

I'm not afraid of death now, and I had resolved my conflicts with my children through our forgiveness ceremony. I had started to understand why I was afraid and why I was afraid to draw the lines. Suddenly the fears start dropping away. And you can't lie anymore. And I'm not young anymore and I'm realizing, "This is who I am." . . . All that gave me courage to stop pretending. I feel like it gave me the courage to acknowledge what I wanted. . . . I never knew what the hell I wanted.

Melanie wanted to go back to painting, and in spite of the financial success of her work, she hated the organizational environment more each day, and decided to leave. "Do you know how amazing it is that I can sit here in this room and not be sweating bullets and not be afraid that I'm going to be fifty, alone, and jobless? To really have the confidence. There are no guarantees. The outside is the same—even less secure—but I am so sure I can handle it. I'm not going to go through my life being afraid. I can't live my life like that."

How we live is a reflection of who we are. Melanie had to begin to live more in keeping with the best image she had of herself. Taking risks is never easy, but Melanie had not given everything away. She had good experience, had kept good friends, taken courses, and saved money. She had just become so busy that she lost sight of an essential aspect of herself for a long while. "The pilgrim's soul is still there. . . . Now I will try to do my art. Will I succeed? I have no idea, but I have some *kochas* [strength] left. At fifty, I'm going back to art with gusto."

Melanie's very human story presents many of the components that each one of us faces in relinquishing old ways, reconnecting to the best in ourselves, and moving ahead. She was going through the normal developmental changes of midlife, set in motion when her second child left home and propelled along by her reevaluation of her relationship with Tim. These changes required her to relinquish old ways of mothering and of being with Tim as well as outdated views of herself. She did not try to become young again. At first she tried overwork, but caught herself and stopped. She then began to uncover the lost Melanie, moved into the losses, and did not try to run away from them with drugs or alcohol. Melanie faced and let go of her personal illusions: illusions that she could protect her children and keep them safe in a dangerous world; that she could meet the expectations of others for her to be a superstar in every area of her life; and that she could bend to fit the needs and expectations of those around her. She mourned the illusions and the roles in her life that no longer fit. She reconnected to an inner strength by listening to her own voice and her own judgments; that is why the video camera story is so wonderful. It could happen to any

The Process of Change at Midlife

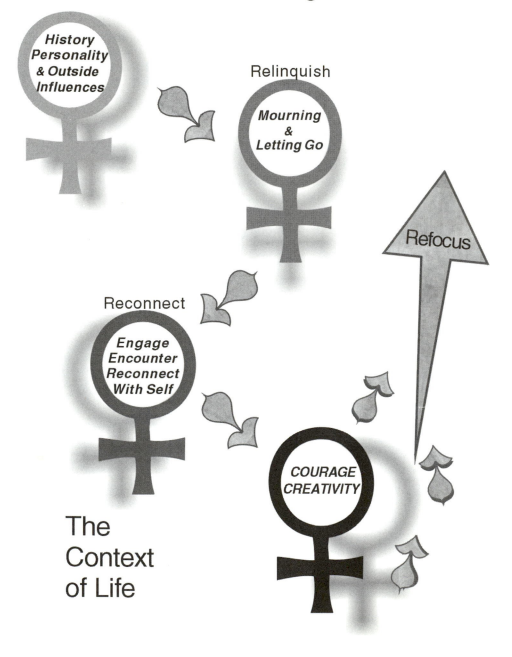

History
Personality
& Outside
Influences

Relinquish

Mourning
&
Letting Go

Refocus

Reconnect

Engage
Encounter
Reconnect
With Self

COURAGE
CREATIVITY

The
Context
of Life

of us. Reconnecting with herself allowed many things to happen. With re-newed confidence, she moved out of the pain engendered by loss, learned to value herself in a way never before possible, and found that she liked herself. These discoveries were greatly influenced by sitting beside her dying friend. Melanie saw the minute difference between life and death in the physical body, and that delicate balance reaffirmed the importance of living fully in the time allotted to her. Melanie gained courage and her fears be-came manageable. Slowly she looked forward, reclaimed her dream as an adult, and went back to painting.

Melanie's creativity is not solely in her ability to paint. Instead, the cre-ativity is in her willingness to find new solutions, new ways to think about life, and different ways to behave rather than endlessly repeating the old ways. This is creativity applied to everyday life—an approach that allows freedom of ideas without immediate censorship of thoughts and wishes, a reorganization of old information into new possibilities, a way to take risks that will enhance life. When she relinquished the old ways, Melanie freed energy that had been bound up. She became more aggressive in her actions when those acts were informed by insight. This energy helped her to take responsibility for her life, to act in her own interest, to get out of excessive caretaking and reactivity, to hold on to a comfortable sense of healthy en-titlement, and to have confidence based on her experience.

As her creative approach to living worked, Melanie gained freedom. Fi-nally, refocused, she took two steps into the dark, left her job, and returned to art full time. Melanie attributed her ability to change to psychological growth, money saved, and support from Tim, friends, kids, and her mother: "people who normally want me to struggle more!"

My dream, right now, is to find a place, find a space that I like, paint, work and come up with a body of work and have a show. I'd kiss the ground if I could have a show and have it be a good show, whatever that means. I would be the happiest woman in the world. Somewhere along the way, since the video camera, I realized that I can do just about anything I set my mind to. . . . So saying that I can do anything I set my mind to is really saying that I'll set my mind to it, and if I don't measure up, I'll deal with that. It won't be my undoing.

The reclaimed self is a powerful and often unexpected resource.

These are some of the themes that I found in talking with women. The women had unique experiences, very different personalities, and diverse lives, but the basic, underlying processes were universal. I have illustrated the way I envision the processes of creative change (see Figure 1). In the pages that follow, different sections of the processes are elaborated with stories and discussion. I blend the actual narratives of women with the psychological underpinnings of each step in this creative process in order to take the mystery, but not the difficulty, out of personal change.

NOTE

Quote in chapter title is from Adrienne Rich, (1981), For Memory, in *A wild patience has taken me this far: Poems 1978–1981* (New York: Norton), p. 22, written when the poet was fifty years old.

❖ 2 ❖

"THE TERRIBLE WEIGHT OF ALL THIS UNUSED LIFE"
Relinquish the Old

So I said to her, "Jane why is it that there's all this unused life?" She just said it was because of men, it was all the fault of men, an' went back to readin' her magazine. An' I thought about it an' I thought, "That's rubbish. . . ." It's not just men who do it to women. Because I've looked at Joe, an' I know it's the same for him. He had more life in him than he could use. An' so he carries all this . . . waste around with him. It's the same for everyone . . . what kills us is the terrible weight of all this unused life that we carry round.
—Willy Russell, *Shirley Valentine*

Judy calls upstairs to say that breakfast is ready, and when she gets no response, she opens her son's door and realizes that he never came home the night before. The same morning, Kate's mother falls and is rushed to the hospital. Down the block, Maria looks around her clean, silent house and wonders what to do until evening.

Our worlds change, so the old roles we have played become outdated. The familiar pictures of ourselves as mother, daughter, and wife fade. Midlife, roughly the years from forty to sixty, requires us to update life in order to feel anchored in the present. How to do that? We review our lives thus far. We modify or relinquish any ill-fitting roles, relationships, behaviors, or self-images. We make practical adjustments to reflect those changes. In these ways, we slowly loosen our hold on the past and feel less encumbered. Not surprisingly, we discover room in our lives where we can emphasize different aspects of ourselves from those we highlighted in earlier times.

When we relinquish the old and connect with the new, we are engaged in a normal, universal process called mourning. The early phase of the process, letting go, is not fun, but is tremendously liberating. Different events encourage us to let go. Aging or children departing are natural occurrences that force us into reviewing life. We rework or relinquish relationships with partners and friends. We sell our house or quit a job; we lose dreams, ideals, or long-cherished images we hold of ourselves or others. With each loss, we are forced to let go, and so we mourn.[1] At midlife, the losses are both concrete and abstract, involving youth and dreams as well as the time left. When our lives are touched with loss, we will grieve those losses that have meaning to us. Failure to let go leaves us stuck.

WHAT DOES IT MEAN TO RELINQUISH THE OLD?

We begin to relinquish the old ways when we have the strength to *face* the aspects of our lives that are changing or need to be changed. Next, we *accept* any losses that occur with change, for example, a husband's anger, a child's disappointment, or the end of a friendship. When we begin to accept loss, we feel the rush of emotions, thoughts, and other internal reactions that accompany letting go. There will be only moments of irritation to mark the small losses, such as the realization that we need reading glasses. But for the significant losses, such as health or relationships, months and years are involved in this intense process of jumbled feelings and ideas that eventually transforms our lives.

When my friend Ellie's father became ill at age ninety, no one was surprised. But his decline made Ellie's mother, who is much younger and physically healthy, so depressed that she stopped functioning as an adult. These changes meant that, in the course of one summer, Ellie went from having two active parents to assuming responsibility for their total care. Luckily, Ellie is an attorney with excellent organizational skills, and she was able to pull resources together that helped her manage the day-to-day responsibilities, but emotionally she fought acceptance of the changes in her parents. Loving phone calls from friends and relatives were little consolation. After the initial dizziness wore off, Ellie felt sad, lonely, and angry. This kind of change, illness of our parents, offers us little. Our goal cannot be to restore life as it was, but rather it must be to accept the reality before us and let go of the past. Losses, especially those that are completely out of our control, are depleting.

Other losses, although equally distressing, are not completely out of our control. Some years ago, I worked with Janine, a vivacious, forty-one-year-old, divorced businesswoman who was having an affair with a married man. Several times a week for six years, this man promised to leave his wife. At first, Janine believed him. But over time, she cycled through disappointment, anger, rage, defeat, hopelessness, fear, and trust in him again. Facing reality took time, but it finally won out over illusion. Psychologically, Janine's struggle was one in which she tested reality over and over again until her belief that her lover would leave his wife ceased to exist. She let go of him and her dreams of a life together. Closing the door on a relationship that could not work was Janine's first step to putting her life back together. It freed her to look for another relationship that had a chance of fulfillment. This loss was not totally out of Janine's control. She could accept the fact that her lover was not getting a divorce and she could control her behaviors, even if she could not turn her lover into the man she wanted him to be. These are two women in very different situations, but both had to face reality and accept the losses they had been dealt.

When our lives are altered in happier ways, we give up little and gain a great deal, but even positive changes require us to leave some bit of life behind. Why did we cry when we graduated from high school? Certainly not because we wanted to stay and take more physics classes. We cried because, although graduation was a success, we were about to leave an important time in our lives and head into an unknown future. We grieve when we are confronted with separations. We feel sad when our children go off to college—not because we want to forever keep them home in their dirty rooms, but because there are certain ways of being a mother that we must relinquish. We cry when our children marry because a profound time in our lives has passed. As we grow, our relationships with people we love undergo alterations. Letting go of aspects of life, even when we want the new life, evokes feelings of sadness and longing. A promotion at work changes relationships with both superiors and subordinates and causes uncertainty. Moving to a wonderful home means that we leave the familiar community and feel anxiety about the new neighborhood. Mixed feelings are natural and healthy. Changes like these are filled with significant gains and usually do not become troublesome, so any small component of loss may pass unrecognized. All the changes described present us with identical dilemmas with respect to relinquishing the old, and we begin in the same ways. We face the aspect of life that has changed or needs modification, and we accept the reality of our situation. As we face reality and accept that our world is changed, we also change; we slowly begin to let go.

How Do We Let Go?

We let go when we loosen the attachment to the person, idea, or dream. Janine gave up the belief that her lover would leave his wife. When she relinquished the dream, she could let him go. Ellie let go of her lifestyle as an independent daughter and became instead the protector of her parents. I have seen letting go happen in many, many ways. It happens with women who want children but cannot conceive or are not married. After many attempts, healthy women let go of the dream. Letting go may mean not having children or it may entail changing direction and giving up the original definition of family by adopting a child. It happens, too, when women realize that they have reached a dead end in love, work, behaviors, and even in ways of thinking. Letting go includes a reluctant and gradual withdrawal of energy, love, and attachment from the person, idea, or dream. Often, we have certain images of ourselves that must be let go. On the inside, we begin to face and accept reality; on the outside, we start to change our behaviors. All the feelings and thoughts occur internally; the behaviors happen on the outside. We let go in idiosyncratic ways.

LETTING GO AT MIDLIFE

In the play *Shirley Valentine*, the heroine has a mini midlife crisis. The trouble begins when Shirley's woman friend proposes a trip to Greece. This offer becomes a major event for the forty-two-year-old, working-class British housewife. Shirley desperately wants to go but knows that her husband will be set against it. Torn and indecisive, Shirley runs into a woman she greatly envied during high school, and this friend confesses that she, in turn, had always admired Shirley. Shirley is shaken into remembrances of her younger, livelier self. "An' then she held my shoulders an' looked at me and said, 'Goodbye Shirley. Goodbye, Shirley Valentine.' (pause) On the way home, on the bus, I was cryin', I don't know why. I'm starin' out the window, tears trippin' down me cheeks. An' in me head there's this voice that keeps sayin', 'I used to be Shirley Valentine. I used to be Shirley Valentine. . . . I used to be Shirley . . . ' (She is crying.) What happened? Who turned me into this? I don't want this."

Shirley faces an unpleasant reality of a misplaced self. The process of change has begun. It starts just like this—with the first inkling of disequilibrium. She reflects on her life, evaluates the last twenty-five years, and begins to grieve. This small encounter sets the wheels in motion, and Shirley decides to go to Greece. Her neighbor Gillian inquires about the trip, and Shirley impulsively lies that she is going off with a lover. Gillian, rather than being horrified, comes to Shirley's house and presents her with a silk robe.

Gillian believed that it was perfectly possible for me to be some marvelous, brave, living woman. I got me mirror out an' looked at meself, an' tried to see the woman that Gillian had seen in me. In Gillian's eyes I was no longer Shirley the neighbour, Shirley the middle-aged mother, Shirley Bradshaw. I had become Shirley The Sensational, Shirley The Brave, Shirley Valentine. An' even if I couldn't see it in the mirror, even if none of it was true about me takin' a lover an' all that rubbish—the point is that Gillian had believed it. Believed it was possible of me. I tried the robe on. It was perfect. It was beautiful. An' in that moment . . . so was I.

Shirley had a glimmer not only of what had been lost, but of all that she wanted to become. All change has two sides. Letting go of the old is only one side. The other side is the creation of space in life for new opportunities.

"I'm goin' to the land beyond the wall. I'm gonna sit an' eat olives on a Greek seafront. An' I don't even like olives. But I might like them in Greece. . . . I'll be Shirley the Brave. Course, I'm terrified really. But I'm not gonna let it show. I'm not gonna let it stop me from enjoyin' things."

No one has discovered a way to escape fear, but Shirley also found courage. Our personalities expand with years of living and feeling. We become tired and sad about what we have done and what has been done to us, so we get angry and take a risk. In Greece, she sits by the ocean and reflects.

What I kept thinkin' about was *how I'd lived such a little life. An' one way or another even that would be over pretty soon. I thought to meself, my life has been a crime really— a crime against God, because . . . I didn't live fully. I'd allowed myself to live this little life when inside me there was so much* [italics mine]. So much more that I could have lived a bigger life with—but it had all gone unused, an' now it would never be. Why . . . why do y'get . . . all this life, when it can't be used? Why . . . do y'get . . . all these feelin's, dreams an' hopes if they can't ever be used? That's where Shirley Valentine disappeared to. She got lost in all this unused life.

Shirley thinks about the life she never led, and her trip to Greece becomes the first step out of being lost. She had put herself in a new situation, and in this space, new feelings and behaviors emerged. She needed courage to tolerate the feelings that accompanied her trip. But the risk paid off. In Greece, Shirley saw herself in fresh ways; mourning is also a process of re-membering all the loveliness in life and in ourselves. She began, for the first time in years, to like herself again. She could never get back to the Shirley of years ago, but she did not want to be a child. She wanted to claim a life as an adult.

At the airport waiting to leave, she asked her well-read, pseudofeminist friend a question that had bothered her for weeks.

So I said to her, "Jane why is it that there's all this unused life?" She just said it was because of men, it was all the fault of men, an' went back to readin' her magazine. An' I thought about it an' I thought, "That's rubbish. . . ." It's not just men who do it to women. Because I've looked at Joe, an' I know it's the same for him. He had more life in him than he could use. An' so he carries all this . . . waste around with him. It's the same for everyone . . . what kills us is the terrible weight of all this unused life that we carry round.

She decided not to return home, and explained to a confused and accu-satory husband, "The only holiday romance I've had, is with meself Joe. An' . . . an' I think . . . I've come to like meself really.' I said to him, I said, 'I think I'm all right Joe. I think that if I saw me, I'd say, that woman's O.K. . . . [S]he's alive. She's not remarkable, she's not gonna be there in the history books. But she's . . . she's there in the time she's livin' in."[2]

Shirley came alive again. In order to be "in the time she's livin' in," she had to make the journey not to Greece, but to a reconnection with her own self. She had to face and grieve the portions of her unused life before em-barking on the rest of it. Shirley reminds us that some of life's most difficult losses are not concrete, like death, but exist without a form, inside, such as the loss of hopes, dreams, or an "unused life."

THE EMOTIONS OF LETTING GO

As we let go, we involve ourselves in an emotional, transformative process that moves us through our loss. Our feelings are unreliable. We move through indistinct stages, going forward and backward, and emotions surprise us all along the way. We need time to adapt to change. Initially, we deny change and loss, particularly when we have been shocked: a husband announces that he wants a divorce, we are told that we have an illness, or we learn that the promotion is not ours. We need time to believe. Ellie was stunned by the rapid changes in her parents, and it took months for her to feel she was on firm footing again. Shirley was more prepared, because internal, developmental changes gave her more warning. But even if we ignore the first signs of change and go along as if nothing is different, awareness eventually hits us, and the feelings begin. When change is major, we can experience physical as well as emotional reactions, such as sickness, nausea, or bodily aches. We can feel beaten up or punched in the stomach. Sleeping and eating difficulties are usual. Whether change is gradual or sudden, there are continuing waves of sadness that shake us as we comprehend that indeed the change is real. Early in the process, Ellie and Janine hoped that things would get better. Ellie hoped her mother's illness would reverse itself; Janine hoped her lover would see all that he was losing. We search for answers, blame, anything to hold on to. Our feelings ride up and down depending on whether we focus on the losses or on the hopes. The longer we focus on the positive qualities of a situation, the longer we remain in place.

Our initial reactions give way to the longest phase in the work of relinquishing the old—the struggle of holding on versus letting go. The emotions change and often become more intense. We have no idea who we will be or what will remain when the process ends. We feel frightened, confused, and unready; some women feel angry, very angry. The anger tells us that we have begun to acknowledge the change. Janine went through confusion, sadness, depression, guilt, fear, and then anger, until she slowly began to face life without her lover. The anger that Janine felt toward her lover was a sign of the realization that they were not ever going to be together. She went through endless lists of what she could have done differently, and she rebuked herself and him. It is usual to feel angry at our own inadequacies, but eventually sadness and depression set in. If we are unable to allow ourselves to feel sad, we remain trapped in anger. Shirley was sad about her unused life. She looked at the dull present, compared it to the lively past, and wanted to let go of all that was sour.

We each have to figure out what aspects of our lives in the past can be kept and what aspects must be relinquished in order to go forward, to become the person we need to become. We must allow all our emotions, shame, fear, anxiety, emptiness, and more.

We are not the same women in our forties or fifties that we were at twenty-five. We may relate to people differently now. We do not love our children, friends, or families less. The women interviewed for this book, and most others, value relationships above all else, including successful careers, but they feel the urgent need to adjust relationships in order to keep them vital. Mothers find it difficult to let go of children as emotional youngsters who depended on them to understand, absorb, and forgive all outbursts. But now we are each more than a mommy, and they are more than children. After a recent argument about the car, I blurted out to my daughter Jenny, "We are both too old for this." She understood and agreed. Moms have to grow up, too.

HOLDING ON TO DREAMS AND LETTING GO OF ILLUSIONS

Courage always plays a role in letting go, but never more than when we face and relinquish the illusions that govern our lives. Recently, I codirected a day-long women's workshop, "Midlife Transformations: Courage and Creativity."[3] A discussion ensued about the difference between illusions and dreams, and in trying to illustrate the distinction between the two, I described a true scene from years ago, when I dropped a towel in the hall, left it lying on the floor, and stepped over it. Later, seeing the towel still there, I asked myself why I hadn't picked it up. And the embarrassing answer was that I wished my mother would do it for me. At the time I was in my late thirties, had been married, had had children, had been divorced, was involved in a career, *and* my mother had been dead for several years. Behaving as if my mother could take care of me was an illusion! Writing this book was a dream, difficult but possible. There are mundane reasons why we need to let go of illusions (they get us nowhere) and why we must reconnect to and hold on to dreams (they guide us).

Illusions Hold Us Back

Diane relinquished her illusions through addressing a seemingly unrelated problem. Diane was forty-two when she began therapy, and she said immediately that she was married to a man she loved but was having an affair with another man who was more exciting and more emotionally connected to her, and she did not want to give him up. Diane's husband of sixteen years had been a good friend to her and an excellent father to their twin daughters, her family liked him, he had been very kind during her mother's long illness, and Diane loved him. But she did not want to give up her lover, who provided an intensity and intimacy that she and her husband lacked. She wanted both men.

Ultimately, in choosing between her husband and lover, Diane had to face the loss of one of the men she loved. That was reality. She also had to give up the illusions of forever being young, of having no limitations placed on her, of believing that everything was possible and still ahead of her, and, in marriage, of believing that she could meet all her husband's needs and he could meet all of hers. These are illusions not easily given up. Diane remained stuck for a long time because she fought against accepting the reality of her situation. It was decided for her when her lover moved away. His departure forced her to ask questions of meaning and learn more about who she was and what she wanted. In spite of her behavior, Diane wanted a happy, intimate relationship, but that meant that she and her husband had work to do together to see if they could build their marriage into an adult partnership. Diane balked at accepting real limitations, but there are other women who prefer limitations and shy away from freedom.

Flora, now forty-four, had a grand summer wedding before her senior year of college, had a daughter right after graduation, and was widowed by a freak accident shortly afterward. She worked as a teacher for several years, remarried, and had two sons. Her husband Keith was involved in setting up a business, so she stayed home to run things when the children were small, and when they got older, occasionally substituted at the neighborhood school. Keith's software company prospered, and the children had the routine skirmishes with grades, cars, and each other. When Flora reached forty, her daughter was in college, the boys were very independent, and she felt out of work. Everyone encouraged her to do "her own thing," but that made her feel worse. Her children had been her "thing" for all of her adult life. At first she protested that they needed her. She was frightened at the impending shifts. Later she realized that the children and Keith were not keeping her captive. She had choices. That did not mean that she *had* to stay home, go to work, go to school, or start a business. Choice meant that Flora, reacting to no needs or wishes other than her own, could knowingly select and commit to a course of action. Freedom can be frightening.

Relinquishing illusions and creating dreams has happened before in our lives, but now, in the middle years, it is necessary again. We have achieved some dreams, we recognize other wishes as illusions that hold us back, and we let them go. We are accepting ourselves and our lives, not passively, but as women fully engaged in our own lives. It does not mean that we love every aspect of our personalities, our bodies, or our families. Reality can disappoint us, but it is a healthier place to live. When we are able to see situations clearly rather than idealizing or devaluing them, we gain a healthy detachment that encourages confidence. Idealizing people or situations misleads us because it causes an exaggerated estimate of other people's potential, based more on our wishes than on facts. Devaluing also misleads us, but in the opposite direction. For example, instead of experiencing envy that a friend was able to spend a month cruising the Pacific Islands, we put down the friend, the trip, or the man she went with. Devaluation understates our feelings to protect us from envy and discomfort. Neither extreme, idealization or devaluation, allows a realistic appraisal of situations we face. Letting go frees us to see ourselves, our situations, and our loved ones without distortion; we can stop blaming and begin blooming.

THE FACTORS INVOLVED IN RELINQUISHING THE OLD

There are universals in letting go, but we are also unique individuals. The situation is like the color wheel; there are only three primary colors, but the combinations are endless. To understand any mourning process, we must know the elements, because the combination of these factors, like colors, creates a unique picture. The most important components are as follows: first, each of us as an individual, including our unique *personality and history*; second, *the loss and the meaning of that loss* to us; and third, the *context and circumstances* of life. These factors dictate our experience of change and create the intensely personal experience of relinquishing the old (see Figure 2).

The stories of two women I have worked with in therapy make these different ingredients easier to understand. Nan, who came to therapy at age forty-one, illustrates the roles that history, personality, and uniqueness of the loss play in creating the process. Nan's history contained a close relationship with her parents, although her mother had died two years before and her father's health was failing; an early marriage and painful divorce; good friends; and devotion to her three children. Although she was very successful—and stressed—as a commercial artist, we talked little about work and a great deal about relationships. Why had she come into therapy? Strange—she was going to remarry and was terrified about the effect that marriage would have on her relationships with her children. None of her children wanted her to remarry, not even her oldest daughter, who was about to go to college. The children wanted no intrusions into the family they had carefully reassembled over the years. Not every family would be upset about remarriage, but this issue was very real for Nan.

Her personality explains more about her discomfort. Personality includes basic temperament, characteristic styles of relating and adjustment, and an integration of our psychobiological systems in a way that makes each of us unique. Nan's mother had been overly protective, and their family had been small and tightly knit. Nan fought to give her children that same protection but within an expanded world. She had worked hard to keep them close after the divorce, and feared that remarriage would destroy her connection to her children. She needed to readjust the relationships with her own children and open the family to include a stepfather. Her parents had been married for thirty-five years. *Her* mom was selfless, *her* mom put everyone first, but Nan saw that her mom also became bitter in her old age and

Factors Involved in Relinquishing the Old

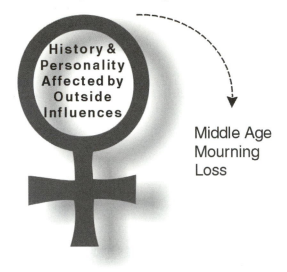

History &
Personality
Affected by
Outside
Influences

Middle Age
Mourning
Loss

The Context and Circumstances of Loss

resentful of some of the sacrifices she had made. There was much about her mother that Nan wanted to copy, but certainly she did not want to repeat the rancor. Nan felt selfish. She dredged up feeling bad about her failed first marriage, although in truth, she regretted the divorce only because it hurt the children. Nan began to feel that she was going to have to choose between her children and her lover. Either decision was guaranteed to make her miserable.

The second element is the particular loss and its meaning. Each loss is different, and each has a distinct meaning. Nan's losses were all abstract. She lost the expectation that she would never have to disrupt her children's lives again; she was reminded of the old sadness that she would never have the *Leave It to Beaver* marriage she had envisioned. She lost the belief that others would protect her as her mother did, and she had to give up her family as it had been and create a new one. Nan also lost the illusion that she could always shield her children, and had to give up selflessness as an ideal and begin to learn about self-interest. Another woman may not have felt the loss, and remarriage would have had a different meaning, but Nan's sadness and confusion were activated by this change—and a supposedly happy one at that!

The third element includes the context and circumstances of life. Context refers to the setting in which change occurs. The circumstances include all the facts or events that influence the experience. For example, Martha, lovely and soft-spoken, was also a woman I worked with several years ago. At the time, she was forty-two and had a good job, friends, and two children. But Martha's husband had just announced that he wanted a divorce after almost twenty years of marriage. Martha's circumstances contribute to the meaning of this loss. She wanted her marriage to continue. She had gone back to work only a few years before and had not progressed very far up the company ladder. Until her return to work, she had been home with one child who needed extensive care after an automobile accident. Her income was one-fourth of her husband's salary, their home was far beyond her means to keep and probably impossible for him to support in addition to a second place for himself, almost everyone in their circle of friends was married, and she had had a mastectomy two years before. Our lives are each embedded in a larger context. For Martha, these realities made the divorce a unique experience and increased her suffering.

As an important aspect of the context, outside influences give additional meaning and provide resources. Imagine Martha facing the prospect of divorce in two different contexts. Suppose she had an inheritance coming from her father; a new medicine had been working wonders for her child's head injuries; an old boyfriend, now widowed, called when he heard the news of her impending divorce; her family and friends rallied around her; her children took the news well; she lived in a town where many others were divorced; and she had already been invited to a support group. Alternatively, suppose Martha's husband had left town with their bank account, she was a devout Catholic who did not believe in divorce, she had just moved to a new town where no one ever got divorced, her family was a thousand miles away, her friends were not calling, and her daughter became so upset when she heard the news that she cut classes for a month and was about to flunk her junior year of high school.

Outside influences and resources include all the contingencies mentioned and more—everything from how-to books to therapy, support groups, friendships that confirm our experience, family members, money to purchase help or ease changes, and religious teachings. Society, too, puts meaning on our life changes. Is it really all right to stay single until you are forty? Is it acceptable to be childless? Change careers? Go back to the world of art given up years ago because you had had to make a "real" living and support the family? Have something to offer outside the home? Be a sexual, powerful, adult woman rather than a perky, charming, young woman with potential? We are greatly helped if the messages we receive from family, friends, and society support our right and ability to make choices, develop ourselves, and engage with our communities in new ways. We are uniquely fortunate if someone encourages us to flirt with danger, question the status quo, and take some risks.

RESOLUTION AND FEELING GOOD

How is relinquishing the old resolved? People often ask me questions like "When will it end? When will I be over it? When will I be back to the way I used to be?" End? Mourning does not end in the same way that a toothache ends. It is part of a process, and we change, we feel different, we feel better. "Over it?" Relinquishing something is not a hill. We go through it, not over or around it. "The way I used to be?" Never. When we truly mourn, we are transformed. We go forward and continue as aspects of life are shaken, dismantled, and rebuilt, until our readjustment is firm.

One of the benefits of grief at midlife is that we have lived; we have amassed enough experiences and made enough mistakes to know a great deal. We have to trust that knowledge to guide us as we recreate our lives. Many of us are finally able to give up the illusion of doing it all perfectly and hoping that all the connections in our lives will be smooth and easy. We are able to replace these illusions with new visions of ourselves that are satisfying. Mourning is a twofold process. It unties us from all that is dead, outmoded, or ill fitting in our lives and reconnects us to all that is living, vital, and authentic. All that we learn during the process, all that we give up and all that we gain, becomes a part of us, and we are enriched. We pass through the empty space and begin to create the new. Our identities are more complete; that is some of our growth.

TRANSFORMATION

Transformation during our middle years comes about as we work through childhood illusions and losses. In the middle years, our sense of ourselves is not derived from self-deception or a desire for perfection, but is born from knowing ourselves and our value. Successful change gives us increased confidence in our ability to untie ourselves from the past rather than feel persecuted by old losses or mistakes. As we begin to look at situations through a deepened awareness and self-realization, we can cultivate genuine values like wisdom, fortitude, courage, a deepened capacity for love and affection, and human insight—qualities that come from an integration of our strengths and shortcomings.[4] We can reflect on the pleasures of relationships and savor tasks that we mastered. Losses are mitigated by positive, loving experiences.

We keep memories and internal images of the past, but these become integrated into our ongoing, forward-moving lives. We are rewarded with two gifts—an alliance with the past and a life in the present. We compromise. That is what adaptation is ultimately about. Not surrender, not triumph, but compromise. Authentic lives are those in which we incorporate all our experiences and reinvest our energies in today and tomorrow. After we have relinquished the old, outdated ways of thinking, doing, and being, we are brought to the final stage of mourning, a creative reorganization of our days. As the process nears completion, we are able to embrace new people, ideas, activities, and work. We establish a new equilibrium. We are increasingly free to create the rest of life with intention and responsibility. If we reach our dreams, we are thrilled; when we fall short, we are proud to have taken the chance. So often we feel that we have lived accidental lives; midlife can change that feeling. This is a time of promise.

We will examine more of these successful struggles and the resulting creative changes in pages to come. If this is the process of letting go, what is it that we specifically relinquish at midlife that will allow us to move freely ahead?

NOTES

Quote in chapter title is from Willy Russell, (1988), *Shirley Valentine*, in *Shirley Valentine and one for the road*. London: Methuen Drama.

1. Sigmund Freud, (1957b), Mourning and melancholia, in *Standard edition* 14: 243–58 (London: Hogarth Press). Original work published 1917.

2. Russell, *Shirley Valentine*, pp. 13, 22, 30, 33–34, 35.

3. One of a series of workshops that focussed on different topics of women's development, codirected with Dr. Nancy Newton in Chicago, 1994.

4. Elliot Jaques, (1965), Death and the midlife crisis, *International Journal of Psychoanalysis* 46:502–14.

"GLOWING COALS UNDER GREY ASHES"
Midlife

One hundred years ago, most women were dead by 45, so I figure everything after that is a second chance.
  —Julia Twomey

One is not born, but rather becomes, a woman.
  —Simone de Beauvoir

Old age ain't for sissies.
  —Bette Davis

"Many—far too many—aspects of life which should also have been experienced lie in the slumber-room among dusty memories; but sometimes, too, they are glowing coals under grey ashes," wrote Swiss psychologist Carl Jung, describing the middle years.[1]

Midlife is a rare segment of life when we are able to see both behind us and ahead of us with a measure of clarity. We can see where we came from and what we have done. We can also see where we are going. Looking either way, we have years of adventures. Knowing that the days to come will be heavily influenced by today, it becomes important to protect an interval of time in which to examine and evaluate our lives, to look behind and release all that is finished, to look ahead and set our plans and attitudes in place for the balance of life. Adult development refers to the changes in psychological structure that occur due to involvement in adult events such as intimate relationships, reproductive choices, work experiences, selection of friends, decline and death of parents, and awareness of one's own mortality. Adult development is built on the past; in that way, it is historical. New structures emerge; in that way, it is also groundbreaking.[2]

WOMEN'S MIDLIFE HAS BEEN IGNORED

The largest segment of the American population is between forty and sixty years old, but midlife has been a remarkably understudied time in the lives of women, although men's "midlife crisis" has been documented for years. Midlife transition was a term coined in a scholarly 1965 article[3] and later adopted wholeheartedly in popular accounts, such as Daniel Levinson's book *Seasons of a Man's Life*.[4] Why have the middle years of women escaped similar attention? Five reasons, at least.

First, midlife refers to the later parenting or postparenting years, and not too long ago, that was a brief span of time in women's lives. The highest mortality rates in this country were for childbearing women and infants. In 1920, the average life expectancy was 54.1 years for the general population. That lifetime would have placed midlife at only twenty-seven years of age! Presently, a woman's life span is almost eighty years. The concept of the "middle years" is somewhat relative, usually defined as extending from forty to sixty years of age, but influenced by socioeconomic class, ethnicity, and race. Upper-middle-class individuals say that middle age starts at fifty years old, whereas women from lower socioeconomic classes feel that middle age begins at forty.[5]

The second reason that women's midlife studies have been nonexistent is that for most of the relatively short history of the field of psychology, researchers have studied boys and men and then made the faulty assumption that whatever was learned about men's development could also be applied to women. Certainly, there are many ways in which men and women are similar, but there are also significant ways in which we differ, and psychology is just beginning to take these individual differences seriously.

Third, researchers have been men and have wanted to understand their experiences. The study of women's issues has waited for women to enter the field in sufficient numbers, with enough clout, to create a body of work.

Fourth, the middle years for women have been ignored because these years have not been considered a positive time. Cultural stereotypes still insist that women peak in late adolescence, when they are most fertile and stereotypically most attractive to men. To feel good about the middle years, women have to believe they have something to offer beyond youthful physical attractiveness.

Finally, two of the major trajectories used to track lives and note milestones like midlife have been chronological age and the course of work. But this tracking system does not work as well for women's lives as it does for men's. Chronological age marks psychosocial changes easily in men because their paths, particularly work, have greater clarity and fewer interruptions, but major transitions occur with more variability in women's lives.[6] Women's lives are notable for commitments that are interrupted and must be refocussed. Transitions become less definable because women are influenced not only by work and age but by having had children or not, being married or not, children's and husband's development, illness, careers, and other responsibilities that may speed up or slow down the occurrence of traditional middle-age issues.

MIDLIFE AS A TIME OF GLOWING COALS AND GREY ASHES

In the past, the middle years were described as terrible because of rebellious adolescent children, crises, divorce, empty nests, fading attractiveness, depression, aging, menopause, and responsibilities for aging parents. But as women tell their own stories, they report something different. Research refutes the starkness of these dramas and finds that children are being launched with a sense of accomplishment, life at home is simpler, and energy is freed to be directed to a partner, work, interests, or one's self. Important, too, during these years, is the fact that income reaches a peak.[7] Writer Joan Mills said of her midlife insights, "I'd gone through life believing in the strength and competence of others; never in my own. Now, dazzled, I discovered that *my* capacities were real. It was like finding a fortune in the lining of an old coat."[8]

THE TASKS OF MIDLIFE

All periods of life have distinct tasks or psychological mini-crises that are expectable and healthy aspects of growth. The crises have some predictability but are influenced by outside forces, previous life choices, our idiosyncratic personalities, and how well we have mastered the life issues that faced each of us earlier.

The tasks vary with each stage of life. For my one-year-old neighbor Corey, the appropriate mini-crisis was trust. Because he was well cared for, he learned to trust his parents, in spite of the fact that they have gone on vacation, frustrated his wishes, or occasionally misread his signals. In adolescence, the work is separation. When my daughter Keira was sixteen years old, she strongly resented being my "baby," relinquishing that protection as she made painful attempts to separate, because she knew that she needed to grow up. At forty-five, photographer Isabelle began to take risks because she realized that life was finite and must not be squandered. Trust, separation, and mortality are issues that we face throughout life, but they become more and less urgent at different times. We do not separate only as teenagers, nor do we deal with questions of trustworthiness only as infants, but at particular times of life, those crises are at the forefront of the emotional work that we do. The better we address each particular issue, the freer we are to move on.

Letting go is inherent in certain midlife tasks and allows old aspects of life to be relinquished. When we can accomplish this, we are free to create the rest of our lives centered on who we are. Whether we feel the middle years beginning in our late thirties or in our fifties, there is work to be accomplished during this time; certain changes are on the doorstep *now*. Isabelle's odyssey captures the tasks of midlife.

Isabelle's Midlife Odyssey

Isabelle described her steady, continued growth through adulthood until more urgent change pressed her as she entered her forties. I interviewed Isabelle when she was forty-seven, at her home late one evening when her busy schedule allowed some time. She was barefoot and in jeans, but glamorous. Isabelle had two children and a full-time career teaching photography. At the time of our interview, she was setting up a new house because she and her husband of twenty-three years had divorced in the past year. On top of this, she had begun a new career as a writer. Isabelle described the gradual shift in her life:

When I think about how my life has progressed, it seems like I've had lots of big changes in the last five years or so, but it's not like . . . I woke up one day and I said to myself, "I don't like this," and I switched directions. That may be the way it can look, but from the inside that's not how it feels. The inside feels much more as if the origins of the changes in my life—that those origins are based in fifteen or twenty years ago. I think that my life has been a steady change, is always changing.

Isabelle recognized that the directions taken and choices made in the past shaped more recent major changes.

In my forties, I have become impatient with some things that I wasn't impatient with before, and I felt that I was going to die someday. And that day was not as far away as it once was, . . . not that death is imminent, but that I could imagine no longer living. I am in good health but it just seems like the days were not to be squandered anymore, that things had to really be on purpose and for purposes that were not just immediately okay, but that really meant something to me. [In the past] it seemed like I was willing to do things that didn't have sufficient meaning, like they were on the next step for me to do. I went to college because you just went to college. I got my first job because, well, I needed to pay rent.

Isabelle's decisions, like choices we all made in our twenties, were based on having endless amounts of time.

I was out of college for a year and worked and discovered what I really loved to do, which was photography, and went to graduate school in photography. And went with the idea of being a commercial photographer because that was the only kind of occupation I knew that made money in photography, and I needed to support myself. In graduate school, I developed an interest in fine art photography, which doesn't pay enough money to support yourself, so when I came out, I did a series of different kinds of jobs and developed a career as a fine artist and began teaching part-time and then began teaching full-time . . . and ended up really caring about it and liking it and developed my career as a fine art photographer, and that was going along swimmingly, but I found that more and more I really enjoyed the teaching. I think I could have been teaching typing. It helped to be teaching something I loved, but what I really liked was the experience of being with people, people who want something and sometimes they're unsure of what that is, people who need to learn the pleasure of discipline and craft and intensity of work. All of those things I liked and still like. And I never thought that I would develop as big a fine art career as I did.

Isabelle beautifully described the gradual change, influenced first by youthful life events and later, increasingly by maturity. The changes continued when she had children, and Isabelle's life took on an importance that it did not have before.

An image that I have of my son when he was just very, very little, a waking image, was of my life being a piece of white paper and this little bitty infant tearing it into pieces and throwing it in the air and it raining down; and it was both scary and beautiful because that was really my life. It was all disordered. It was so hard to work everything out in terms of time. But the main thing that I was having trouble dealing with was not the time but if I was going to do this at all, I wanted it to be important. So I started to shift.

The changes that Isabelle felt sped up. "I shifted what I did and started documentary photography, which was about real things in the world, real people, and not what I had been doing. And that was the beginning of something I really see happening now in my life, so my work had to become more significant to me, and that meant taking on a social tone." Isabelle's last big project was "trying to take very realistic portraits of people with AIDS . . . that their humanity would be sort of undeniable, and it's really the first portraits I ever took, trying to engage their presence . . . really careful, studied work."

As her children got older, she made more serious changes in her life.

But now in my forties, . . . I realized that I was in a marriage that didn't mean anything to me, and that I disguised that for myself for a long time because everything else I liked a lot. I liked my professional life, I liked being a mother, and I liked the idea of being a married mother in an intact family. I finally realized that, again, I'm going to die someday. And I don't want to die having lived my life like this. Those are the big changes. They are all stairsteps of the progression.

Although the middle years bring certain general issues to all of us, we can see how choices that we made earlier or choices that were made for us will have an impact. Isabelle became a mother in her middle thirties rather than in her twenties. Life became more serious with children, and that influenced her view of photography. She could not tolerate squandering her days. Other women are propelled into an evaluation of life through their own unique circumstances.

Isabelle's story illustrates the major tasks of midlife and some of the optimal outcomes that are possible. The tasks can be examined through the

Midlife Losses

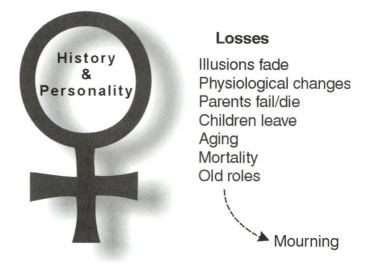

Losses

Illusions fade
Physiological changes
Parents fail/die
Children leave
Aging
Mortality
Old roles

Mourning

changes, gains and losses, that occur in three overlapping clusters: physiology, attitudes and roles, and acceptance of mortality. All the tasks at midlife require us to relinquish aspects of youth, but they also offer adult compensation. First, we will examine the losses (see Figure 3).

Physiological Changes

The changes in physiology include declines in youthful sexual attractiveness, physical strength, intellectual functioning, and fertility, and menopause. Even Isabelle, who still turns heads, commented, "Of course, I get very irritated that shop clerks won't notice me because I'm not twenty-five. I'm just hitting my prime and you're not paying attention to me now?" Our prime internally occurs later than the outside prime time.

We are accustomed to our bodies changing; we are already familiar with hormonal shifts because we have felt them with our menstrual cycles, with pregnancies or attempts to become pregnant, with nursing, and with menopause. Therefore, changes associated with aging, although unwelcome, are not shocking.

Time begins to run out if we want children or more children. There is the diminished capacity to get pregnant. We know the odds of carrying a baby to term change as we age. For women who have waited to have children, the desperation sets in no matter how trendy it is to become a first-time mother after forty. Renee stopped the fertility treatments after two years and adopted a child; Leslie married a man who her friends insisted was no different from all the other guys she had dated because it was time to begin a family; Liz gave up trying for a daughter and started a new business; Susan's husband had a vasectomy because the pain after each miscarriage had become unbearable. Isabelle, divorced at forty-seven, with two children, said, "I haven't gotten to the end of wanting children," but childbearing decisions are made by our bodies without our consent. That door is closed. Even with the miracles of assisted pregnancies, we ultimately face the end of childbearing. It is a natural ending.

Physical changes become apparent at midlife. We notice a reduction in physical strength; we have to work harder to maintain physical well-being. Muscles are strained and body parts need to be stretched. Weight is easier to put on and harder to take off. Eating habits need revision, again. We understand that cholesterol is bad even though we had never heard of LDL when we were younger.

Other physiological changes bring concerns about intellectual functioning. K. Warner Schaie studied intellectual abilities in more than five thousand adults and maintains that it is difficult to confirm general intellectual declines prior to age sixty. There is no uniform pattern of age-related changes in all intellectual abilities; instead, declines are in specific areas.[9] Researchers identify fluid intelligence as the dimension that falters. Fluid intelligence is our ability to effectively respond to very novel problem-solving situations whose solutions are out of the context of what we already know. Problems inherent in aging, such as illness, diminish our abilities to integrate novel information. We tend to lose flexibility and openness to thinking in totally new ways, so we perform more poorly on measures of fluid intelligence. Also, illness and lack of stimulation foster deterioration, so any restrictions on lifestyle work against us.

Attitudes and Roles

The second cluster of tasks in which we experience losses involves growing up and taking charge in new ways. These tasks include an acceptance of adulthood and different types of responsibility, the ability to live in an "empty nest," adjusting to different forms of nurturing, and an examination of successes and failures.

We let go of the idea that other people are the grown-ups; we are the grown-ups of the generations in our lives. This recognition brings a heavy sense of responsibility.[10] My parents died, one shortly after the other, when I was thirty-five. I was divorced and had no family nearby other than my young daughters. My parents had always been there, and then they were gone. I felt chillingly alone. Strangely, my younger daughter, who was only five at the time of my parents' funerals, turned to me and said, "Everyone move up one seat." I asked her where that comment came from, because she echoed exactly the way I felt. It was from *Alice in Wonderland*, as Alice was pushed around the table at the Mad Hatter's tea party, waiting her turn to be beheaded. Feelings of responsibility increase with the loss or aging of our parents because the buffer between us and old age is gone. Mature adulthood has negative aspects because it means the decline of the generation that has gone before us, the people we have relied upon, and those who have taught us and provided guidance.

Many women assume the care of aging or ill parents during the middle years, and that responsibility has the potential to become exhausting because the demands and losses are so much more obvious than the joys. All the work goes toward slowing down the inevitable.

Somewhere along the way, we lose that sense of forever being seventeen. Not that we feel old; the word chokes me, but we feel not-young. Simone de Beauvoir wrote, "One day I said to myself, I'm forty. By the time I recovered from the shock of that discovery, I had reached fifty."[11] Youth is gone, childhood is irretrievable, and there are funny hairs growing out of our chins.

We assess our lives and count up the mistakes and failures in all areas. We remember naive, silly mistakes and times we listened to other people when we should have listened to ourselves. We remember major errors that have caused pain and slowed us down. Midlife becomes a time when we are intensely aware of limitations and failures. If we worked, we worry that we missed out on personal relationships; if we did not work, we regret that we were not tested in the outside world.

The empty nest has moments of sadness. Children keep us firmly attached to life. Meals, laundry, homework, and car pools have an unmistakable reality. Holding a child in our arms keeps us grounded and reminds us of what is important and what is irrelevant. All the mothers I spoke with had no doubts about the value of active mothering and were certain about the importance of the job. When the nest empties, we do not feel as needed as we used to.

Mortality and Last Chances

The third cluster of tasks involves the confrontation with personal mortality; we begin to believe that someday we will die. Therefore, we experience a growing sense that we face last chances. The loss is that we feel the emptiness of not having taken certain roads if we have not led the lives we wanted. We become pressured, more than we have ever been, to make choices. Experience, health, and time are exhaustible. Therefore, choices that we make take on a seriousness and a finality. Is there time to do all that we have planned and hoped? Midlife is a time when some individuals (so far, only men) become president but many others are given early retirement.[12]

Just as a burial brings a death into consciousness, confronting mortality makes us aware of all the limits, from our own petty inadequacies to those on a worldwide scale. We face these little deaths that occur regularly in our lives, like the disappointments in our children, husbands, friends, and in ourselves. We stop beating our heads against these walls or we are doomed to leave these decaying remains lying around where we poke at them every once in a while to see if they are gone or if we can resuscitate them one more time.

Midlife offers compensation for the losses we experience (see Figure 4). In each cluster of tasks, there are "glowing coals under grey ashes."

Adjustments in Midlife

Adjustments to Physiological Changes

Midlife offers restitution for physiological declines. Not one of the women I interviewed or read about expected to be exempt from aging. Instead, they developed a healthy and creative attitude toward adulthood. The women turned inward to nurture qualities that are not depleted but are enriched with time and experience.

We are able to give up some of the self-consciousness of youthful sexuality without giving up sexuality itself, we attend to our bodies, and we develop creations that are not babies. Because enjoyment of sexuality is enriched by experience, connectedness, and comfort with our bodies, sexuality remains as possible as ever. Midlife offers opportunities to nourish relationships in ways that were more difficult in young adulthood when external messages of "should" rang loudly. Isabelle noticed the difference: "It is a wonderful thing about being in your forties. . . . At the same time there is increasing invisibility that women get as they get older, interpersonal relationships are not at all a problem."

Researchers now agree that intellectual ability declines later in life than previously thought, and declines are smaller and involve fewer functions. One important type of intelligence, crystallized, continues to grow even into late life. Crystallized intelligence refers to a fund of stored knowledge and the ability to draw upon and apply that knowledge to current situations. We keep increasing our knowledge base and our ability to draw on it. There are

Midlife Compensation

Letting go leads to - - - - -

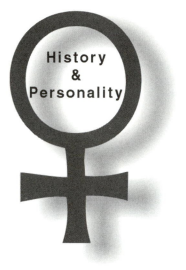

History & Personality

Gains

Adult dreams
Self-care
Generativity
Children launched
Productive work
Time
Confidence
Courage
Experience
Assertiveness

many lifestyle factors that influence intellectual functioning. Good health, favorable environmental circumstances such as money, education, career, or being a member of a well-functioning family all help our intellect. Lifestyles that include complex tasks and stimulation, opportunities to learn and think, responsibilities, independent judgment at work, reading, or travel provide activities that help us maintain intellectual flexibility and performance in middle age and beyond.[13] Numerous studies remind us that adults who take advantage of cultural resources continue to develop intellectual abilities.

Women who possess broad interests adapt well to the demands of old age. In a study of more than two hundred white, middle-class men and women, it was the group of working, middle-aged women who remained engaged in life, showed the most concern about social problems, and participated in activities. The women were not spectators; their lifestyles involved family and a wider range of social activities than the other people studied.[14] Community is essential because it is within a social structure that we, as mature women, continue to adapt.

Physically, there is no doubt that the firm bodies and easy health that we once took for granted now must be protected and attended to, but middle age provides the sophistication and confidence to experiment with alternative medicines, meditation, and other less conventional ways of feeling healthy and attractive. For some women, self-care means finding time to delight in more conventional ways of feeling good! The generations reaching middle age now may have been educated, but they are not particularly pampered women. Joan, a businesswoman who has three daughters, said at forty-six, "You know, I never had a manicure until I was in my forties because my life was filled with important things like the kids and work. I want to try a few self-indulgent things—do things that I have always wanted to do but never had the time—go to a spa or take a ceramics course."

I know what she means. Both my daughters have encouraged me to "chill" on numerous occasions and, although it is good advice, it does not come easily after years of hard work. In the middle years, it dawns on me that I have led a serious, meaningful life so far, and I ought to try some nonsense in the next portion.

Adjustments in Attitudes and Roles

Attitude and role adjustments are very positive and liberating. Parenting changes but does not end, as the nest empties. The portion of our brain that was endlessly filled with information about the kids—where they were, how they were, the time we were supposed to pick them up, questions about whether we were ruining their lives or they were ruining our lives—has space for other thoughts. We can relate to our children differently when they are on their own. Even if they are "not what we ordered," as a client who is a writer aptly phrased it, we loosen our beliefs that we have to guide them, support them, and anguish over their mistakes. We can enjoy them, or not, as the adults they are becoming and respect their right to make mistakes and suffer just like we did. Barb said, "Now I'm defining my territory." She and her husband bought a second home and she "wants a family spot for [all five] children to congregate, but no kids just dropping by." In the past, she could take time for herself only when she was worn out and desperate.

Areas in which our own growth had been thwarted can be reopened when we see our children able to take risks. They encourage us to be brave because when we see them experiment successfully, we are often freed to try new things. We learn from our children all through the mothering years, but in midlife, the children are usually launched or getting ready to leave home, and our worries, even as they naturally continue, are tempered by the knowledge that our children have their own lives to lead, just as we do.[15]

Adolescents and young adults, having adopted our values and dreams, may carry shared dreams further, out of healthy identification with our values rather than out of burdensome attempts to correct our failures. Some of our interests are shared by our children. I have noticed that psychology never appealed to either of my daughters as a career, but both are naturally insightful, take this gift for granted, and bring it to all work. Carrie, a music teacher, never got any of her three children beyond perfunctory music lessons, but they love to attend performances together. Other interests are our children's alone, and we follow them. Our worlds are broadened by learning about their passions, and our relationships with them are transformed into more mature connectedness.

Responsibility for our lives, success and failure, and mentoring or caring for others are all linked in the lives of women. The summation of this work can be called generativity. Generativity is a term introduced to psychology by Erik Erikson, a psychoanalyst who spent his life studying the formation of identity. He theorized that we go through eight stages of ego development during our lifetimes. Each stage has a choice to be made or crisis to be mastered. Accomplishing the psychological work of each stage allows us to go successfully to the next. The stages that apply to the second half of life are Generativity versus Stagnation, followed by Ego Integrity versus Despair. Erikson believed that the central development of middle age was generativity, which

encompasses the evolutionary development which has made man the teaching and instituting as well as the learning animal. The fashionable insistence on dramatizing the dependence of children on adults often blinds us to the dependence of the older generation on the younger ones. Mature man needs to be needed and maturity needs guidance as well as encouragement from what has been produced and must be taken care of. Generativity then, is primarily the concern in establishing and guiding the next generation.[16]

When he published that passage, in 1950, it was generally accepted. As I read it today, I recognize that he described the lives of middle-aged men, not women. Being needed can enrich us, as Erikson describes. Having others, older and younger, depend on us can be rewarding, particularly when our guidance is appreciated, but Erikson never fully took into account just how much women care for, nurture, and guide others throughout their lives and the fact that when that is all there is in life, it depletes rather than enriches us. Enhancement of self comes from mutuality in giving and receiving, and an aspect of the middle years is reformulating the balance of these nurturing activities. Women have always been good at guiding the next generation. What has rarely been acknowledged is that, in the middle years, we need to attend to ourselves as well. Generativity, in the broadest sense, is far greater than being "mom"; it encompasses all our creative productions, including creation of an authentic self.[17]

The women I spoke with did not want to be young adults again. At a barbecue last summer, my friend Julie's twenty-year-old nephew impressed himself by telling us stories of barhopping and pickups. He sees us as hip but old, in need of entertainment. We see him as unenviably young and green.

Maturity is fine as long as we find value and joy. Megan was glad youth was gone because adulthood brought greater happiness. Just married for the first time at forty-three, she said, "I wanted to grow up. I [wanted to] accept responsibility for my life, be in charge of it. Accepting intimacy on that level. That level of closeness . . . I wanted that responsibility. That was being in charge of my life." Claire had a similar experience when, at fifty-two, she opened her own business consultation service. She recalled how afraid she had been in her twenties and into her thirties, thinking everyone knew more than she did. "Now I listen to myself more closely than I listen to anyone else. Sure, there are limitations in middle age, but for me there were also limitations, *big ones*, to being young."

Years ago, a group of exceptionally gifted children were studied. The women from that group were reinterviewed when they averaged age seventy-seven, and findings showed that these gifted women had careers *and* were homemakers for most of their lives, at a time when careers were not as common as they are today. Researchers also found some interesting differences between the more creative and less creative women in this gifted group. The more creative women had engaged in more activities outside the home after age forty-five than the less creative women. They felt generative and were happier, but not healthier psychologically, than the less creative women. As they aged, several of the creative women had increasingly escaped from societal inhibitions and, after the age of sixty, had done amazing things, such as editing a newspaper, publishing, or performing music.[18] What we see is that at midlife and beyond, generativity appears in creative ways that go beyond the care of others and into business, relationships, and artistic productions.

When the women I interviewed were honest with themselves, they saw that they were ready to take charge of their own lives and wanted validation for all they knew. They had become increasingly comfortable with their own set of values, and these beliefs gave them a secure base from which to venture out. Midlife women have much to offer, and begin to recognize that fact. Finally, we are able to take credit for what we do and what we know. After fifteen years of running a successful development staff, one woman realized, "I really advanced people. I gave people breaks." She had taken time to train and mentor people. "I'm proud. . . . I have been a good role model and have tried to manage them with a human, nongossiping [touch], none of that male pee-on-every-wall thing."

Generativity involves responsibility for guiding the next generation, although that does not necessarily mean our own children. Generative activities afford us creative ways of living in the middle years and beyond, not doing the same caring behaviors over and over, but discovering new forms of creative living. There is not one way to be generative, or even one way that works for our entire lifetime. Different forms of generativity work better at different life stages and in different circumstances. For example, a thirty-five-year-old mother of three is generative by caring for her children, whereas a woman of fifty, childless or with children launched, can use that generative capacity in other forms, such as mentoring or creative work. The middle years become a time to reexamine our goals and direct our efforts.

Having responsibility is nothing new. What is often missing in women is confidence and power. Responsibility can include reclaiming power and taking charge of our own lives. I link it here to generativity, which refers to responsibility for others, for the future. Without generativity, the middle years and beyond become empty. With only generativity and no responsible interest in our own lives, we become so entirely other-focussed that we grow estranged from ourselves.

The middle years are traditionally a time of productivity in work, so if there is more that we hope to accomplish, this is the time to begin. Many standard definitions of success have been thrown at us; we need to pause and create a personal definition of accomplishment, whether it includes work, children, relationships, integrity, authenticity, health, survival, or other values. Success in this second cluster of tasks neccesitates an adjustment in attitudes and roles. An optimal outcome is our achievement of a new balance of attention to self while still giving to the larger social community. We have time to pursue a stimulating life, which mitigates the losses of aging. Erikson stresses the need to take our place in society, develop and perfect all productions, and accept responsibility for our creations. This means that we take risks, concede to disappointments, and relish successes.

Accepting Mortality and Last Chances

The days are not to be squandered, so we develop an increased awareness of the preciousness of the moment, an ability to live in the present, and a willingness to overcome vulnerability and take risks. Many of us retain adult, personal goals that need to be examined and pursued so that we do not suffer lowered self-esteem from failing to live close to our cherished ideals.

Central to all midlife tasks, perhaps at the source, is an increased awareness of life as finite.[19] Generativity in the deepest sense comes to the fore in the middle years because we have become aware of limited time to live. It has been suggested that Americans still seem to think that dying is optional, but historian Robert Jay Lifton has a less cynical view. He believes

our knowledge that we die pervades all such larger perceptions of life's endings and beginnings. And our resistance to that knowledge, our denial of death, is indeed formidable, as Freud and others have emphasized. But that denial can never be total; we are never fully ignorant of the fact that we die. Rather we go about life with a kind of "middle knowledge" of death, a partial awareness of it side by side with expressions and actions that belie that awareness.[20]

Having this "middle knowledge" contributes to our sense of looking at our last chances. The recognition of last chances leads to the opportunity to use our time well. By now, we have full, rich histories and can use our memories of the past as a guide to solving problems of the present.

With the birth of each of her four children, Karen had taken a few weeks off and then headed back to her work as a radiologist in a suburban New York hospital. At forty-five, she quit her job, and shortly after, explained that "here's my last chance to be home and do childcare full-time when Sara's at kindergarten." Sara is her fourth and final child. If Karen wants to be a full-time mother and she passes it up now, there will be no more chances. So her choice took on a now-or-never quality. She had always felt that her education and special training demanded that she work. With that attitude, Karen's degrees burdened her rather than liberated her. But now, like other midlifers, Karen wanted to use her time differently, in a role she had never fully allowed herself. She compared the way she had lived to the way she wanted to live; she understood the mistakes she had already made and did not want to repeat them. By making those comparisons, she clarified her values and was able to create a life closer to her wishes to spend more time enjoying motherhood.

Realizing that life is finite raises questions of ultimate values. The women I interviewed, like many others, were inspired by a phoenixlike creativity to affirm life.[21] When we come to terms with being mortal, we think about what is important to us, and often we are more willing to be guided by our values.

We pay more attention to the *processes* than to the *products*. The process is the essence of work. The ideas, creations, or productions are not themselves the end products, but are rather the starting points and may be reworked, modified, and elaborated upon, sometimes for years. We can sense this dynamic going on in Isabelle's life; as her life changed, her work went from fine art photos to documentary work and eventually to writing, in an effort to move closer to the heart of life issues. She had begun to feel that she was stranded on the surface with her photographs.

Mortality makes us confront the ultimate limits of life itself. Early adult idealism relies on our denial of two fundamental features of human experience—eventual death and the existence of hate and destructive impulses in each person. Our young adult naiveté allows us to live within the myth that we, through good intentions and will power, can right the wrongs of the world and of others. Life, with expectable mistakes and failures, naturally challenges these myths. At midlife, we have the opportunity to give up naive idealism. We are challenged to accept the fact that hate and destructive forces are fundamental to our own nature, although not at the expense of inherent goodness. Our experiences can reassure us that the balance between love and hate tips to the side of love. Damage is healed by loving grief, envy is softened by admiration and gratitude, and confidence and hope come from knowing that losses and grief can be endured and overcome.[22] Intimate knowledge and acceptance of our own limitations can provide a basis for genuine compassion for others.

On a very personal level, acceptance of limits means that imperfection no longer need be felt as bitter, self-persecuting failure. Midlife demands acceptance of the fact that we cannot achieve all we had hoped and planned. We cannot even hold on to all we have achieved. We can resign ourselves to accept the inevitable frustration of life. It need not be experienced as a personal indictment.[23] We can shift from impatience with ourselves and others to a more reflective and tolerant stance. The drive to perfection can be lightened by knowing that, as humans, we will inevitably make mistakes. The lessons of maturity and reality can motivate us toward goodness rather than toward perfection. This deepened sense of reality provides more synchronicity between who we are and how we act. We can become more whole.

Acceptance of personal mortality often evokes the healthy search for continuity and transcendence beyond our individual lives. It can drive us to make connections, to find continuity in what has come before us and what will come after us. Transcendence speaks to our connectedness to all life. Immortality can be expressed in different modes: biological, theological, natural, experientially transcendent, or creative. Biological immortality is universal and emphasizes generational continuity, children and grandchildren. Theological immortality is seen in religion, although not necessarily by a specific life-after-death belief. Many people construe theological immortality as love or energy that continues beyond death. Natural immortality refers to nature itself, the belief that the natural environment will always remain. Experiential transcendence refers to the psychic state many mystics describe, in which time and space disappear.[24] Creative immortality certainly can be great works of art, science, or literature. Fundamental to transcendence is our attitude toward our own lives—an attitude that seeks new forms and expansiveness; continuity through living fully in work, service, or care; and moving toward psychological wholeness.

When we heal ourselves, we transform our piece of the world into a better place. Thus mature work in many forms does not have to impoverish us but can be brought back inside, stimulating a cycle of creativity. The external creation is experienced as life-giving, not sapping. By creating from this source, we can regain a sense of wholeness of ourselves and others that is not false or idealized. Artistic or not, menopausal or not, with or without children, the middle years are special ones for women. If we forget to attend to ourselves now, the biological clock, because it stops, can remind us to preserve these years for living. We must shelter days to *be in time* rather than to *pass through time* paying attention only to the endless tasks that have gone before in our lives.[25] The beauty of the middle years is that we are at a place in the journey where we can appreciate engagement in any work or play as an expression of our productivity and creativity. In that way, we prepare for the personal losses of old age and eventual death by actually living a bit. In a culture that privileges youth, we must learn to value age. We can enjoy in the present rather than live only with memories of the past or dreams of the future.

NOTES

Quote in chapter title is from Carl Jung, (1971), *The portable Jung* (see note 1).

1. Carl Jung, (1971), The stages of life, in J. Campbell (Ed.), *The portable Jung* (New York: Viking), p. 12. Original work published 1931.

2. Maureen Murphy, (1992), Psychoanalytic treatment at midlife, *Psychoanalysis and Psychotherapy* 10(1):61.

3. Elliot Jaques, (1965), Death and the midlife crisis, *International Journal of Psychoanalysis* 46:502–14.

4. Daniel Levinson, (1978), *The seasons of a man's life* (New York: Ballantine Books).

5. David Chiriboga, (1981), The developmental psychology of middle age, in J. Howell (Ed.), *Modern perspectives in the psychiatry of middle age* (New York: Brunner/Mazel), pp. 3–25; Bernice Neugarten, (1968a), The awareness of middle age, in B. Neugarten (Ed.), *Middle age and aging* (Chicago: University of Chicago Press), pp. 93–98.

6. Barbara J. Reinke, (1985), Psychosocial changes as a function of chronological age, *Human Development* 28:266–69.

7. Valory Mitchell and Ravenna Helson, (1990), Women's prime of life: Is it the 50s? *Psychology of Women Quarterly* 14:452.

8. Joan Mills, quoted in L. Clark (Ed.), (1977), *Women women women: Quips, quotes, and commentary* (New York: Drake), p. 15.

9. K. Warner Schaie, (1994), The course of adult intellectual development, *American Psychologist* 49(4):304–13.

10. Helen Meyers, (1989), The impact of teenaged children on parents, in J. Oldham and R. Liebert (Eds.), *The middle years: New psychoanalytic perspectives* (New Haven: Yale University Press), pp. 75–88.

11. Simone de Beauvoir, quoted in Carolyn Heilbrun, (1991, Summer), Naming a new rite of passage, *Smith Alumnae Quarterly*, pp. 26–28.

12. Meyers, The impact.

13. Schaie, The course; Steven Roose and Herbert Pardes, (1989), Biological considerations in the middle years, in Oldham and Liebert (Eds.), *The middle years*, pp. 179–90.

14. Marjorie Fiske Lowenthal, Majda Thurnher, and David Chiriboga and associates, (1975), *Four stages of life* (San Francisco: Jossey-Bass).

15. Meyers, The impact.

16. Erik Erikson, (1950), *Childhood and society* (New York: Norton), pp. 266–67.

17. Linda Edelstein, (1997), Revisiting Erikson's views on generativity (paper presented at the 104th Annual Meeting of the American Psychological Association, Chicago, IL).

18. George Vaillant and Carolyn Vaillant, (1990), Determinants and consequences of creativity in a cohort of gifted women, *Psychology of Women Quarterly* 14: 607–16.

19. Elliot Jaques, (1981), The midlife crisis, in S. Greenspan and G. Pollock (Eds.), *The course of life*, vol. 3, pp. 1–23 (Washington, DC: U.S. Department of Health and Human Services).

20. Robert Jay Lifton, (1979), *The broken connection: On death and the continuity of life* (New York: Simon & Schuster), p. 17.

21. Jaques, The midlife crisis.

22. Lifton, *The broken connection.*

23. Jaques, Death and the midlife crisis, p. 513.

24. Jaques, Death and the midlife crisis; Jaques, The midlife crisis.

25. Lila Kalinich, (1989), The biological clock, in Oldham and Liebert (Eds.), *The middle years*, pp. 123–34.

❖ 4 ❖

"First It Was in Black and White, and Then It Was in Color"
Creativity and Insight

Every blade of grass has its angel that bends over it and whispers, "grow, grow."
 —Talmud

Imagination is the highest kite one can fly.
 —Lauren Bacall

Creative minds have always been known to survive any kind of bad training.
 —Anna Freud

It is never too late to be what you might have been.
 —George Eliot

It isn't a sin that we are in the dark room. It's just an innocent situation, but how fortunate that someone shows us where the light switch is.
 —Pema Chödrön

The speaker at a commencement ceremony I attended recently turned to the graduates, threw open her arms, and exhorted them, "Embrace change!" Being told to embrace change is like being reminded to exercise and eat healthy foods. We know it is good. We just cannot stick to it. Asking for a new view in the middle years opens the door to "embracing change." This chapter describes the attitude of creative thinking that helped women actually act on this desire.

Change requires us to dismantle and rebuild. Creative thinking is an essential instrument for change. It allows us to freely play with new ideas and approach the world with openness and enthusiasm. Creative thinking allows for novel ideas and insights that lead to new ways of being and doing. We do not need to be talented or extremely artistic to think creatively. It is an everyday approach to life, not a one-time production. Many of the women

Creative Thinking

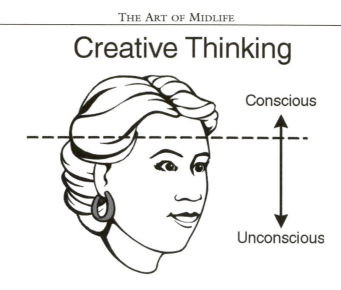

Conscious

Unconscious

I interviewed were naturally imaginative; others learned to allow creativity to emerge.

There is no mystery to understanding the creative process. In the story that follows, Ann describes the insights she achieved and how she actually felt. Other sections of this chapter examine how creative thinking is related to individual personality, the connections between creativity and psychological health and illness, and some real obstacles that exist for women who want to cultivate creativity in their lives.

THE PROCESS OF CREATIVE THINKING

Creativity emerges from processes that exist between our consciousness and our unconscious (see Figure 5). Therefore, creativity is influenced by both awareness and unawareness, and all that is available and unavailable in conscious thought.[1] It requires an openness to all of our thoughts, feelings, and reactions. In certain states of attention, like that between sleeping and waking, the barriers we generally have against new ideas are temporarily permeable. Thoughts and feelings that are usually unacceptable or out of our awareness flow freely back and forth, so ideas that we might have censored can be reached more easily than under other conditions. Forces that usually hold back ideas now bring them forward. Openness to this more fluid state of mind can be frightening. Insight often happens in moments of transition or during relaxation, because we are less vigilant then.[2] We have all had new ideas or insights occur in the shower, in the car, or even watching television, because there is less self-scrutiny at these times.

We confront anxiety when we create. We feel the temporary nothingness when we question what we used to believe without clarity about what we will believe. I used to feel these sensations often when I was in the middle of my own, lengthy psychoanalysis. Now the anxiety strikes when I write. My analysis somewhat prepared me for the fear that precedes new ideas and the struggle to entertain them. The work becomes worthwhile because of the delight that accompanies the breakthrough of an idea that is new to me.

When we are not overly burdened by fear and guilt, preconscious processes make free use of symbols. Our minds mix dissimilar ingredients into new patterns. We reshuffle experience and awaken to new ideas. Recently in therapy, Joan and I have been discussing her healthy and reasoned decision to end treatment. Joan is thirty-nine, works in insurance sales, and came into therapy for anxiety attacks and relationship problems. As she has become increasingly self-aware, she has also become more confident and curious about understanding her feelings. She walked into one of our sessions very angry. She described her irritation and persistent bad mood, but she had not been able to find any causes. Suddenly she looked at me and said that all week she had been pursued by the memory of an event from twelve years ago. "I had bought my first car and, on my way to work, smoke came out of the hood and it broke down. They said it needed $400 of work. I asked my parents for a loan because I had left Dick and had the baby, but my parents said no. I had to junk the car." What did this memory mean to her? That her parents had abandoned her and left her alone, without help, over and over again. Then the lightbulb went on, she giggled, and we brought the memory into the present and connected it to feelings about leaving therapy after so much work together. With freedom of thought, the feelings and ideas that at first seemed like apples and oranges settled into meaningful patterns. Preconscious processes contribute to creativity when we feel free to gather, assemble, compare, and reshuffle ideas. Gathering and reshuffling is a form of free association during which the mind "shakes itself apart and together again, finding its way off the beaten path, stumbling onto new connections."[3] When we are creating, our minds move without conscious deliberate bias or preconception from thought to thought, idea to idea, or feeling to feeling. We do not choose ahead of time to think or talk about any particular topic or restrict ourselves to a topic when one comes to mind, so we have an endless supply of old data rearranged into new combinations (see Figure 6). We enjoy increased freedom in how we think about the minutiae of living—thinking, walking, talking, dreaming— and indeed of every moment of life.[4] Instead of feeling only the limits, we experience spontaneity. But spontaneity requires a lack of self-consciousness, which can be difficult for women. We tend to be overly aware of others. At first, this way of thinking can be frightening because of the strange and random thoughts that emerge. As this process becomes comfortable, the creative thoughts or insights become an anchor to feeling whole without outside help. We learn to rely on this process, and it provides us with a

Rearranging Data into New Combinations

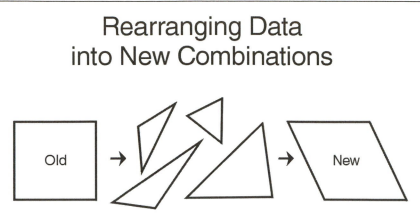

guide. In therapy, too, where thoughts and feelings that have been long hidden are allowed to emerge, these processes occur. Creative thinking reconnects us, in this way, to buried aspects of ourselves.

When we freely roam our mental highways, unhampered by stoplights and stop signs, we are thinking creatively. We gather bits of seemingly unrelated ideas and impressions, put them together in varying combinations until new patterns are formed. We reorganize available information into new forms; we uncover "what has always been there."[5] Of course, there is the brand new idea, the new fact, but most writers agree that the highest form of creativity is the ability to approach the old ways from a different point of view. "What characterizes the genuine creative act is not the addition of novel information, but the use of new programs for processing the already available information."[6]

There is a second part to creative thinking. After we form a new pattern, we step back. We subject our ideas to self-critical scrutiny for the necessary, mature, secondary process of checking and testing.[7] When the first phase, the free flow of disassembling and reassembling, gives way to the second, more conscious phase, the creative thinker steps back from her work and becomes an observer. She views what she has done from the outside. Groups and companies have made good use of the knowledge of creative thinking in "brainstorming," which deliberately separates the formulation of ideas from the evaluation of them. In the first phase, everyone is encouraged to share all notions, even silly ones. Others respond and build on them. No judgments are allowed. Only later are participants allowed to critique, evaluate, and select ideas to be used.

When we observe the creative process in others, we are often struck by the unconventionality or independent judgment and forget that discipline, endurance, and tolerance are also integral to creative thinking. This process sounds very solitary, and much of it is, but creativity is also attuned to others. It is not completely isolated, although there are periods of introspection that are very internal. As in brainstorming sessions, the input of others can push us to be more open. What we learn from new ideas also can connect us to others in healthier ways. When the women I spoke with made changes, they were not trying to disconnect from people. Instead, they were often trying to improve relationships. Some women saw the changes they made as a result of facing broken aspects of themselves or their relationships and a desire to build ways that would work better.

INSIGHT: ANN'S STORY

Insight is born from the process of creative thinking. It is when we relax that the areas we are most intensely struggling in become illuminated. We are aware of the focus we put into problems and feelings, yet we continue to be surprised when our insights fall into those areas.

Ann is a thirty-nine-year-old, married hospital administrator. She is tall, apparently fearless, direct, and very likable. When she told me about her out-of-doors exploits, I wasn't surprised. I had known her for a while, and when I told her about my book project, she said she had a story.

Ann had been adopted from an orphanage when she was seven months old. It was no secret, and her parents' delight at having her was always evident. Another child had been adopted after Ann, but had died in childhood. When Ann was thirty-eight, her mother died, and Ann grieved intensely. Shortly afterward, she decided to begin a search for her biological mother.

So then I called the adoption agency and it turned absurdly easy. I thought this was going to be a mythic quest, but basically, you give them a hundred and twenty bucks and that's that. I do remember that I was on the waiting list for six months before I got the legal documents [to begin the search]. Then I decided absolutely that I wasn't going to do this—this was going to open something that I was really very scared of. It was only after I had been in therapy a significant amount of time that I started feeling fear. I never let myself be afraid, *ever*, in my life. I used to do technical cliff climbing, rode motorcycles; I pushed that probably more than I should have. But [now] I was enormously afraid, and that is a feeling I am not used to dealing with.

I spent an hour staring at these [legal documents] and decided I *was not* going to do this, not going to do this. And then I did it. I did it because somewhere I had an instinct that I wanted to get better and no amount of therapy would do that, no matter how good my marriage would be, no matter what. The only other way would have been to somehow confront some of these issues with my mother, but she was no longer alive. One of the things I had paid for was a condensation of my [birth and adoption] records. I got really scared of what that would say. It took a long time to come. I started getting scared of lots of things, but it was all related. I joked that I would put it in a safety deposit box and not open it; if it came, I couldn't be in the same house with it. . . . Well, it came and it was real ordinary—what nationality I was, brothers and sisters, religion of parents, one page. I realized when I read it, that what I had been so scared of was that I came from nowhere. I know that is totally irrational, but my experience had been nothingness and I translated that to, "I came from nowhere," so when I read this stuff, half of what I needed got healed by that. There was objective proof that I came from somewhere, and those people were traceable. It seems very strange to me when I talk about it, but it was very much that way.

This is insight. All the thoughts and feelings about where Ann had come from had been buried for years. Her mother's death, therapy, and working on problems broke up the blocks inside. She reshuffled her experiences and had her startling revelation. When this breakthrough into consciousness occurred, Ann was confident that it was true. There was no other way. When insight occurs, we often wonder why we were so stupid not to have thought of it earlier, but we were not ready. We were not yet open to knowing.

Ann decided to go further and search for her biological mother, although when she found out her history, much of her work was done.

Usually these searches take four years. A week later, they found her! I wasn't quite ready. . . . The paper coming convinced me that I came from somewhere, so the rest was fine. . . . The first letter I got from [my biological mother] was really nice. It wasn't scary. . . . Then I talked to her on the phone for the first time, on the first of June. You pick up the phone and dial ten digits and there you are. It was like eating birthday cake.

When I talked to her, at least that first phone call and everything since then, has been partly a process of mutual reassurance, as in "I'm not mad at you for giving me up and I'm not mad at you for looking me up."

There were more insights for Ann. After she received the letter and knew she "came from somewhere," she realized that she had never allowed herself to think about the seven months before she had been adopted.

To make speculations about [my biological mother] was absolutely taboo. Totally. I never allowed myself. I didn't develop a picture in my mind. That was absolutely walled off. When my therapist once asked me if I had ever thought about looking for my birth mother, I thought I could have handled it a whole lot better if she said to me, "Have you ever thought about sleeping with your father?" [To ask about looking for my birth mother] was a really awful thing to say, to even imply. Can you imagine how much psychic energy that took! Not thinking. Not at all, until I saw that document. That was why it was so healing.

Ann had clues to her secret before this insight, because she had the same strange experience each time she sat in her therapist's waiting room. "I was sure that the person who opened the door was not going to be her. I was terrified of that. I would sit in the waiting room hunched over, and when she would open the door, I couldn't look because I was sure it would be somebody else. She would forget. This is too weird!"

Ann's fears told her two important facts—she, who rode motorcycles and scaled cliffs, was thoroughly terrified of talking because it would reveal her secret, and she feared that people who were important to her would disappear and be replaced by strangers.

The decision to search was connected to her adoptive mother's life and sudden death. Ann's mother had never consciously stopped her from looking for her birth mother, but it took her mother's death and the subsequent terrible grief to open the door. "I was enraged at my mother for dying as she did [suddenly and without warning]. So I think I may have [unconsciously] said, 'Screw you and your taboos.' If you can do this to me, see what I can do. That was some part of the motivation. What I had always been scared of happened." Ann's mother had promised that she would never leave, and then she did.

Ann's father told her that in his discussions with her mother, her mother had been fine about the possibility of Ann searching for her birth mother. "I don't know if on some other level, or I just made it all up [that I wasn't allowed to think about my birth mother] but I don't think that at the age I developed that taboo, which was pretty young, . . . I could have developed it on my own. I think she was a part of it. I think that her grief at not being able to have kids translated into the taboo for me."

Ann felt her mother's grief at being unable to conceive and dealt with it by obliterating her birth mother and the seven months prior to her adoption. One result of obliterating those months was this terrifying, nameless belief that she came from nowhere. "I wished through the whole process that mom was alive so I could talk to her about it. I think I would have [searched for my birth mother] anyway, because it was the remaining issue between us. I would have forced the issue, and I believe she would have responded."

I knew that Ann had functioned well socially and in her job; she was bright, healthy, and happily married. I asked her if she had known what she was looking for, what she needed to heal. "There was nothing in the outside world that [not knowing where I came from] stopped me from doing." But since finding her birth mother,

there is an enormous amount that I do differently. For instance, I used to never cry about anything. I cry [now]. It's fine. What I used to believe about change was that it is a long, slow, incremental process. But it was a process of accumulating. I changed like this (snapped her fingers). I was a much different person . . . in forty-five minutes [after reading that document containing my history] . . . that's the way it feels. Remember *The Wizard of Oz*—at first it was in black and white, and then it changes into color. That was me inside. It was all there before, but suddenly it was in color. It was like blood went through my veins.

I came from somewhere and I met the someone. And I don't have to hide that anymore. That was always a fear, that if you were in a relationship with me, if you knew me too well, you would find out my awful secret, which was, "I came from nowhere. I started at seven months." Not that I was adopted.

It's amazing what becomes one woman's secret. "It's so irrational, and I think of myself as a rational person. I never would have told anybody that because *I never knew it myself. I only knew it when it was gone!* It was such a relief. I read this document, looked up, and said, 'I came from somewhere. I really came from somewhere.' "

This insight had an effect on other aspects of Ann's life.

Before, I always felt, in any of my relationships, that I was a fairly minimal part, and now I don't think that. Now I think I'm an important part of a relationship, for some people more than others. Somewhere along the line, after this, I realized that I'm the sort of person that people like, and I have qualities that people like. I never, ever believed that prior to this. I think that is a function of being given up. If your mother can give you up, what faith is there that anyone else can't and won't? My parents provided as stable a home as possible, but I had a brother that died young, and we moved, and that contributed to instability. I know the world can change quickly.

I have more faith in other people. Even if we never saw each other again, now I have some faith that you would have some memory of me. Before, I would have said that is utterly impossible.

This also meant that Ann learned how to leave rather than waiting to be left.

I was supposed to be given up, but I couldn't leave. I had a role. I think I am an equal partner in a relationship now. I can leave—or I can stay—but I'm not dependent on your decision. Before, I had to be utterly dependent on your decision because . . . I didn't have the capacity to make that decision. My role was to be given up. I have as much of a right as the other person. I'm free. The worst things that can happen have happened to me, and the best things that can happen have happened to me. I have wondered if this is the adventure of my life. But if it is, then how do you live the rest of it? If it continues like it has, it has been wonderful. I look forward to living. I used to wish I was eighty and could look back and see how it turned out. Now I'm loving living my life. All this great stuff is now accessible to me. I'm living free, and there is a lot to be said for living free.

As frightened as she was, Ann trusted her internal processes to guide her. That is a difficult path for some women, particularly if their experience has been discounted in the past. Ann trusted the irrational, trusted the unknown and unseen processes guiding her, tolerated the discomfort of new feelings, and was patient. Meeting Ann, one would have had no way of knowing any of this. It was all intensely personal and private. This series of creative insights was a small, but profound, aspect of her life.

Because the insights were profound, they reverberated and caused other changes, not necessarily in behavior, but in attitude. It has affected her marriage—not that she wants to leave, but for the first time, she knows she is able to leave, and that knowledge, without her acting on it, causes discomfort to her husband. Those ripples have not yet settled into a new equilibrium. The last time I saw Ann, she was beginning graduate school with some fascinating ideas for a new career.

THE MOTIVATION FOR CREATIVE THINKING

Why did any of these women need to take risks? Why did they spend time and energy on changes that terrified them? They did so because they saw it as a solution to their inner struggle. They made changes because they were motivated by curiosity, pain, unhappiness, anger, desperation, the urge to find new ways to approach problems, or fears of complacency. We do not change because life is going perfectly. Normal growth is sometimes coupled with pressures such as family problems that intensify internal demands. The result for many women is a spirited surge to take hold of their lives in new ways. The most successful women made creativity integral to their everyday lives. External moves are only geographical; the internal motion must be present for a psychological journey.

There are writers who maintain that both neurosis and creativity, although very different activities, arise from attempts to solve inner struggles. Adaptation to loss is one of the struggles, and creative activity is commonly thought to be a method of self-repair. The creation replaces a lost part of ourselves or of someone close to us. The product symbolizes that lost person, ideal, or aspect of us, and in that way, creativity is healing. There is evidence that an overabundance of artists have suffered grave losses in childhood, usually the death of a parent. For some, their art is an effort to repair damage to themselves; for others, art recreates the lost person. Usually, the loss is twofold; we have lost someone, but when the person is essential to us, we have also lost something of ourselves. Another school of thought maintains that creative work can result from successful mourning of old losses. Sometimes the artistic products that result from mourning even show the issues that figured in the loss. For example, the theme of grieving parents emerged in artist Kathe Kollwitz's work after the death of her two sons. I have noticed, throughout my own life, creativity is connected to separations. As a child, I turned to art when my parents were out of the house for the evening, and, as children tend to do, proudly offered them the painting when they returned, maybe with the hope that the gift would keep them home. This use of creativity continued into my adulthood. My first book, on the adaptation of mothers to the deaths of their children, was written in part to lay to rest my own sense that the world was filled with random events, lucky and tragic. My feelings had lingered from years before, when, as an infant, my daughter Keira survived a terrible two-story fall through the laundry chute in our home, landing in the basement in a pile of unwashed laundry. The actual writing of the present book, too, began with loss, this time Keira's leaving home. Creativity restores a sense of wholeness and completeness. Some call it a sense of cohesiveness and integration, of unity or continuity of the self. In Ann's account and other stories, women describe over and over again that they have been finding their way back to some authentic self, a kind of wholeness that had eluded them and is essential at midlife.

Is creativity self-centered? Yes and no. Yes, because it heals the self. Yes, because it grows out of our need to experience ourselves as complete and unique individuals. Yes, because we must look inward during certain portions of creative work. No, because we offer something new to the world. Creativity is not necessarily for the purpose of destroying the old, although it can do that. Rather it is to repair, renew, and recreate for the benefit of all of us. One analyst disputes the notion that artistic expression is primarily self-love, seeing it rather as a collective love:

It seems unlikely that the artistic performance or creative product is ever undertaken purely for the gratification of the self, but rather that there is some fantasy of a collective audience or recipient, whether this is a real audience, as for the stage, or the unseen audience of the writer or the painter; whether this be contemporary or extend into the limitless future. The artistic product has rather universally the character of a love gift, to be brought as near as perfection as possible and to be presented with pride and misgiving.[8]

CREATIVITY AND PERSONALITY

Personality style influences our tendency to approach problems in novel rather than stereotypic ways. Suz finds one way of doing things and then looks for different ways, while Pat is content to repeat the first solution forever. Suz develops a variety of solutions, which puts her in a better position to meet new problems than Pat, who relies on one solution. Suz is freer. Pat's restrictive thinking keeps her life organized within the same patterns, behaviors, and beliefs. Problems arise when Pat becomes too rigidly bound to previous conclusions because she does not allow in new elements, and thus insight cannot occur. Suz has different strategies, new techniques, and a willingness to try out new ways of understanding her experience. It does not mean that Suz loves change or is not frightened. It means she is less locked into certain patterns of thinking or stereotyped ways of being. Adaptability allows Suz to put aside one pattern of behavior that no longer works and experiment with a different approach. We all approach life in mostly habitual ways. We don't wake up in the morning and look for a new method to brush our teeth, but rigidity and restrictiveness in thought, behavior, and coping styles are reasons why insight occurs less easily for some people than others.

Women who are not flexible can become more so. It is no accident that many of the women I spoke with have been in therapy. Insight-oriented therapy is an ideal place to learn how to examine and reorganize experiences and memories as well as to develop new attitudes and ways of looking at life. We lose the fear of new thoughts. Our minds become trained to stay open to new explanations and solutions. To what extent a woman can change her approach, no one really knows. Certainly, with the developmental personality changes during the middle years, the opportunities are available, but we have to recognize an open door and find the courage to walk through.

Creativity requires us to reach into all aspects of ourselves rather than remain content with stale responses. Carl Jung espoused an interesting notion that buried aspects of personality can emerge at midlife. Emergence of these new qualities can facilitate a creative approach in the middle years.

When Jung was at the beginning of his own middle age, in personal crisis and distressed by the war in Europe, he noted the general reluctance of individuals to address problems. "We wish to make our lives simple and smooth, and for that reason, problems are taboo. We want to have certainties and no doubts, results and no experiments, without even seeing that certainties can arise only through doubt, and results only through experiment."[9] Jung believed that until age forty, most people are preoccupied with meeting obligations that revolve around raising a family and establishing one's place in society, and that women had to focus on the expressive and nurturing facets of their personality.

The nearer we approach to the middle of life, and the better we have succeeded in entrenching ourselves in our personal attitudes and social positions, the more it appears that we had discovered the right course and the right ideals and principles of behavior. For this reason we suppose them to be eternally valid, and make a virtue of unchangeably clinging to them. We overlook the essential fact that the social goal is attained only at the cost of a diminution of personality.[10]

As the demands of family lessen, women are free to balance their personalities by giving expression to the previously suppressed aspects. They can turn toward unexplored qualities that were previously incompatible with the nurturing attitudes and behaviors necessary during the parenting phase of life. Jung wrote that we see a slow change in a person's character, where certain traits may come to light that had disappeared since childhood. In other people, we may observe that previous inclinations weaken, to be replaced by different interests. This direction allows creativity. Unfortunately, there are some people, Jung believed, who harden their convictions and principles, especially the moral ones, until they become intolerant, as if the principles were endangered and needed additional protection.[11]

Midlife is the period when traits emerge that had previously been suppressed in the service of blending us to fit into an ordered society. Jung believed that we accomplish change at this time by attending to our inner worlds. It is necessary to attend to the inner life in order to assure a successful adjustment to the second half of life. A wonderful line from one of Jung's essays reads, "But we cannot live the afternoon of life according to the program of life's morning; for what was great in the morning will be little at evening, and what in the morning was true will at evening have become a lie."[12] We are women of the afternoon.

WOMEN OF THE AFTERNOON

Jung's view that turning inward, or introversion, occurs is supported by others. Sociologist Bernice Neugarten calls a similar process "interiority" and places it later, in the fifties rather than the forties. She sees the forties as a decade in which individuals have high energy and see the world as a place where bold risks are rewarded. Later, there is a movement of energy away from the outer world to the inner world.[13] Interiority includes increased preoccupation with ourselves and our own needs rather than those of others. Jung sees the shift as a result of a change in the psyche and compares it to the sun rising, spreading light and warmth ever wider, until at noon it attains its greatest goal and then begins the decline, which is the reverse of rising—"the reverse of all ideals and values that were cherished in the morning."[14] The rest of the self appears.

Jung compares the components of masculinity and femininity to a psychic storehouse, where unequal supplies of substance are used in the first half, leaving the remainder for the second half. Therefore, women reach into more of the supply of masculine qualities in the second half of life. Jung goes on to say that in youth it is a mistake to be overinvolved with one's self, but the older person, having "lavished light upon the world," must now illuminate herself. He notes how unprepared individuals are for this change and how much confusion is experienced, but reminds us that "whoever carries over into the afternoon the law of the morning . . . must pay for it with damage to his soul."[15] Freeing the repressed aspects of ourselves offers the potential to attain greater personal completeness. Jung made discoveries about himself during his middle years that he continued to sculpt for the rest of his life, reminding us that creativity finds different, satisfying expression throughout life.

Like Jung, writers today also talk about women's midlife ability to reach into the so-called masculine, or instrumental, attributes and integrate these qualities with established expressive abilities so both contribute to work and play.

BLENDING THE MASCULINE AND FEMININE

Results of various studies and women's descriptions of themselves lead to interesting conclusions. Many midlife women are able to use the natural developments of aging in their favor. Sometimes, they learn it is better to be more direct than they have been in the past. Too many of us were raised on the fantasy "Be a good girl, and it will be given to you," a motto that results in passivity during youth and resentment in old age.

Researcher Florine Livson found that women in midlife savor qualities that had been buried in their previously other-filled lives. Two samples of healthy, fifty-year-old women were compared. The women in one group remained psychologically stable since forty; the others had improved from age forty to fifty. The stable women were feminine, gregarious, conventional, and placed a high value on closeness with others. There was minimal conflict between their personalities and their social roles as wife and mother. The second group, consisting of those women who gained psychological stability between the ages of forty to fifty, turned out to be quite different. These women were ambitious, skeptical, introspective, and unconventional. The differences were in personality, not in intellect. The second group of women, called "independents," were more autonomous, less conforming, and more in touch with their inner lives than the traditional women. It turned out, in looking at their pasts, that the differences in these women were apparent from adolescence. The independents felt more stable later in life because when they were younger, they experienced a conflict between their personalities and their social roles. They were less in sync with society. They were, by virtue of their personalities, unconventional but living conventional lives. When they felt freer, at age fifty, they became satisfied. These women had loved their domestic lives and were devoted mothers, but life expanded at fifty—for nontraditional women who had lived traditional lives.[16]

Another study found similar results indicating that creative women show a pervasive independence of judgment that tends to free them from tightly prescribed, culturally imposed sex role behaviors. Creative women struggle less than others with feeling overly dependent or fighting against their dependency. They are neither cold, passive-aggressive women nor superfeminine "dolls," but reject overly feminine and overly masculine traits. Their confidence lets them worry less about threats to their liberated status. They are free to develop imaginative relationships.[17] We can keep all that is good about being feminine and in midlife can add assertiveness and independence of judgment, qualities that have been traditionally viewed as "masculine." This is the best of both worlds. It becomes increasingly possible at midlife because we have access to and feel freer to express more of ourselves. These changes are not losses of psychological characteristics but are expansions of our existing personalities in new directions.

With age, women use emerging independence to increase their skills to cope with life's problems. As a result, we become less defensive and have greater self-esteem. These qualities coincide with greater commitments to work, which begins to equal, but not replace, active parenting. Research concludes that in our forties, women are becoming increasingly the people we wanted to become.[18]

Researchers constructed a typology based on personality dimensions that sheds light on why it is easier for some women to approach the middle years with a creative attitude. The four types were: Individuated, Traditional, Conflicted, and Assured. The Individuated group had the qualities most conducive to creative living. They demonstrated independence, intellectual capacity, social poise and status, and self-expression. For a variety of different reasons, each of the other groups were more inhibited. The Traditional women adapted so well to their surroundings that creativity was lost, but was not felt as a loss. The Conflicted women lacked the social skills and confidence necessary for success. The Assured women lacked the introspection and openness fundamental to creative approaches to life.[19]

Researchers try to figure out what influences our personalities at midlife by studying specific variables. But we have learned that it is neither one factor nor another. The changes we have examined cannot be attributed to menopause, the empty nest syndrome, or involvement in caring for parents, although all these factors make an impact. It is not simply biology or social roles that enable positive shifts. After comparing personalities and different life paths of more than one hundred women, Ravenna Helson and Paul Wink concluded that personality continues to change in adulthood and the shifts reflect long-term trends, not single life events. Personality also evolves due to response to the demands of different periods of life. Interestingly, the years around age thirty and between ages forty and forty-six are reported to be times of difficult transition, but life settles down after two or three years and women find increased emotional stability.[20]

In a survey of seven hundred women between the ages of twenty-six and eighty years, respondents most often described their lives as "first-rate" when they were in their early fifties. When this study was repeated six years later, again it was the women in their early fifties who were most pleased. The women considered their lives first-rate because, among other reasons, they were more their own persons and were able to bring both feeling and rationality into decision making. These women felt that they had developed more control over their lives.[21] We are more in control because midlife is a time when we are less reactive to others' emotions and to our own emotions, and the actions we take are less colored by emotions.

CREATIVITY AND EMOTIONAL WELL-BEING

Twentieth-century United States has incorrectly intertwined the notions of creative and neurotic. This is a recent distortion; artists of the past were not seen by their contemporaries as disturbed, but rather as working people. It seems to have become a common assumption that creative people are crazier than the rest of us and their disturbances are due to their creativity or their creativity is aided by their problems. There is nothing reasonable that supports these notions. Creative and neurotic processes are universal because both arise in early childhood, not out of exceptional circumstances, but out of simple and common human experiences. Therefore, potential creativity is as universal as the neurotic process, but it is not the same thing.

There are links between artists and psychopathology, but it is not that being creative causes emotional instability or that emotional instability creates art. The link is more complicated. For example, studies show that creative artists experienced more emotional difficulties in early life, had longer and higher alcohol use, more use of drugs, and more problems with depression, mania, somatic disorders, anxiety, psychoses, and adjustment disorders and that therefore they used therapy more often.

Different problems seem to appear in different creative arts. More specifically, theater people, writers, artists (but not architects or designers), musical performers, and composers experience more emotional problems as compared to public officials, military personnel, social scientists, physical scientists, and some business people. Women writers describe more depression than nonwriters. Their relatives who were not depressed are also creative.[22] Higher levels of creativity were found in patients diagnosed with manic-depressive illness than in other patients or normal individuals, but their normal relatives also scored high.[23] A 1994 study suggests that mood is related to increased quantity rather than quality of creative production.[24] Other professions show higher levels of different problems, for example, businessmen and entrepreneurs gamble.[25]

Do individuals in the arts admit to more problems? Do they describe their emotions more elegantly or intensely? Do certain problems aid creativity? Are we to assume that creative professions attract those people who are predisposed to certain problems, or is it that creative professions, because of inherent stress and lifestyle, aggravate hidden problems? We find creative individuals in an interesting array of fields. Not surprisingly, artists, such as painters, rank high on tests of creativity, but more interesting, physical scientists and social scientists are also creative and do not rank highly in the realms of pathology. This suggests that it is not a quality of creativeness that distinguishes members of various professions but perhaps the requirements of the profession or the type of creative expression. There are creative people who are healthy, and there are many, many disturbed people who cannot create. Severe personality disturbances will not enhance creative work, but rather will interfere with it.

What motivates creative expression? A twenty-five-year follow-up study of ten women who as adolescents had evidenced exceptional creativity examined their motivation. The women's responses indicated that they sought to satisfy inner psychological needs for: understanding their personal reality, maintenance of order and control, and emotional mastery of their experiences. Understanding subjective reality helps us to be comfortable with and accept our own processes. Establishment of order in our creative productions compensates for our lack of control in the external world. Emotional mastery helps us regulate our feelings, counteract our depression, feel our strength, and maintain excitement.[26] And the motivation that draws us to creative activities is to fulfill inner psychological needs.

Creative women in the middle years were also found to have defense mechanisms, those protective patterns of thinking and behavior, that are among the most mature adaptations possible in adulthood. The women showed very healthy defenses of altruism (the ability to act for others unselfishly), sublimation (the redirection of socially unacceptable impulses into socially acceptable channels), and humor. These defenses help creative attitudes and provide a needed ingredient—the capacity for play.[27]

The implications for women at midlife become clear. Creative thinking helps us feel better and more complete. Creative thinking can anchor us to the deepest aspects of ourselves as our lives shift under us. Disruptions shake us up. In the midst of changing roles, changing bodies, and changing families, it does us little good to try to reestablish life exactly as it was. Creative responses are useful, however, because they permit change while simultaneously holding us firmly to our core. With each creative response, we have a hand in shaping ourselves.

WOMEN AND CREATIVITY

There are two disturbing factors in the creative process that predominantly affect women. First, creativity requires that we allow new thoughts and feelings. Although women are excellent at expressing thoughts and feelings and remarkably tolerant of intense emotion, we do not like the notion of breaking down the old, even to make way for the new. It raises the specter of disconnectedness. To say yes to the new, we must say no to the old.[28] This can become a problem. Many of the women interviewed had waited and waited before taking action. Some waited overly long, until they felt so trapped that it was anger that finally forced them to seek new solutions.

The second dilemma for women is that society does not always want our creations, other than children. This lack of fit between our gifts and society's requests inhibits creativity. Without encouragement or validation, creativity is almost impossible to sustain. In reviewing more than 2,400 Japanese women creators and leaders from 580 to 1959, it was found that when the creative zeitgeist favored literary activity, both men and women were likely to participate. When male aggression and power was in force, women writers were stopped by societal pressures. Sexist ideologies discouraged women in the early years of their personal development and further inhibited their achievement when they matured.[29] Many women have low confidence from being told over and over that their gifts of empathy are useless, their talents are silly, and their experience is invalid. The women I interviewed went back to trusting themselves instead of the voices of well-meaning others who had taken away their experience. It is easier for women who had childhoods where feelings and experience were valued and where imagination and fantasy were enjoyed rather than dismissed. These childhood experiences may help women retain the spirit of play into adulthood. In a *Newsweek* interview, Howard Gardner, a researcher on creativity, noted that it is a peculiar combination of youth and maturity that allows the most revolutionary work to take place.[30]

Society treats women strangely. Virginia Woolf wrote that actual women were quite different from female characters in fiction. The contrast between the two was striking. In books, poetry, and men's imagination, women are valued. "Practically she is completely insignificant. . . . [S]he is all but absent from history. She dominates the lives of kings and conquerors in fiction; in fact she was the slave of any boy whose parents forced a ring upon her finger. Some of the most inspired words, some of the most profound thoughts in literature fall from her lips; in real life she could hardly read, could scarcely spell, and was the property of her husband."[31]

Woolf goes on to note that until Jane Austen's day, women were not represented in fiction as friends, although men had those relationships. Sometimes women were mother and daughter, but usually they were shown only in their relation to men. Suppose, she muses, that men were only represented in the literature as the lovers of women—how literature would suffer.[32]

These dilemmas explain why images of famous, creative women are not tumbling into your mind. Artists had a chance because they had a product to display that might find favor. But even at the height of her fame, Georgia O'Keeffe's flowers were sensationalized as erotic and she was always referred to as "the female artist." To say "female artist" does far more than identify her; it creates a separate category, as do the terms "lesbian politician" or "woman doctor," a category that is different, not in the mainstream, and almost always implies "less valuable than" the main group. In *A Room of One's Own*, Virginia Woolf wrote about the difficulties for a woman who wants to be creative, in this case, a writer. She alluded to women as outsiders and wrote that men have "no need to hurry. No need to sparkle. No need to be anybody but one's self."[33]

Woolf gave advice to her imaginary writer: "above all, you must illumine your own soul with its profundities and its shallows, its vanities and its generosities, and say what your beauty means to you or your plainness." She was exhorting women to write authentically about their own experience, about their own meaning. In examining the creative paths on which the women I interviewed refocussed their lives, I found that they moved toward a more authentic way to be and to live, a way finally possible in the middle years when pleasing everyone else fades in significance as we realize the impossibility of the task.

Virginia Woolf watched her mythical novelist:

I saw, but hoped that she did not see, the bishops and the deans, the doctors and the professors, the patriarchs and the pedagogues all at her shouting warning and advice. You can't do this and you shan't do that! Fellows and scholars only allowed on the grass! Ladies not permitted without a letter of introduction! . . . So they kept at her like the crowd at a fence on the race-course. . . . If you stop to curse, you are lost, I said to her; equally, if you stop to laugh. . . . Think only of the jump, I implored her, as if I had put the whole of my money on her back; and she went over it like a bird. But there was another fence beyond that and a fence beyond that. Whether she had the staying power I was doubtful, for the clapping and the crying were fraying to the nerves. But she did her best.[34]

NOTES

1. Ernst Kris and Lawrence Kubie both wrote on this topic. Ernst Kris, (1975), *Selected papers of Ernst Kris* (New Haven and London: Yale University Press), pp. 473–93; Lawrence Kubie, (1961), *Neurotic distortions of the creative process* (New York: Farrar, Straus and Giroux, The Noonday Press). There are other theories of the creative process, but this chapter relies mainly on the theoretical underpinnings described by Lawrence Kubie.

2. Kubie, *Neurotic distortions*, p. 27.

3. Ibid., p. 53.

4. Ibid., p. 37.

5. Arthur Koestler, (1964), *The act of creation* (New York: The Macmillan Company), p. 120. Koestler wrote that the "act of wrenching away an object or concept from its habitual context and seeing it in a new context is . . . an essential part of the creative process" (p. 529).

6. Pincus Noy, (1984–85), Originality and creativity, *Annual of Psychoanalysis* 12–13:423.

7. Kubie, *Neurotic distortions*, p. 54; Kris, *Selected papers*, p. 485.

8. Phyllis Greenacre, (1957), The childhood of the artist, in *Psychoanalytic Study of the Child* 12 (New York: International Universities Press), p. 58. Noy agrees with Greenacre's description of art as not narcissistic for creative scientists and artists.

9. Carl Jung, (1971), The stages of life, in Joseph Campbell (Ed.), *The portable Jung* (New York: Viking), p. 10. Original work published 1931.

10. Ibid., p. 12.

11. Ibid., pp. 12–13.

12. Ibid., p. 17.

13. Bernice Neugarten, (1968a), Adult personality: Toward a psychology of the life cycle, in B. Neugarten (Ed.), *Middle age and aging* (Chicago: University of Chicago Press), pp. 137–47.

14. Jung, The stages of life, p. 15.

15. Ibid., p. 18.

16. Florine Livson, (1976), Patterns of personality development in middle-aged

women: A longitudinal study, *International Journal of Aging and Human Development* 7(2):107–15.

17. Catherine Bruch and Jean Alston Morse, (1972, Winter), Initial study of creative (productive) women under the Bruch-Morse model, *Gifted Child Quarterly* 16: 282–89; Jean Alston Morse, (1978, Winter), Freeing women's creative potential, *Gifted Child Quarterly* 22(4):459–67.

18. Ravenna Helson and Geraldine Moane, (1987), Personality change in women from college to midlife, *Journal of Personality and Social Psychology* 53(1):176–86. Helson and Moane studied a group of women in an effort to determine personality changes that occur between college and midlife. They found that women at age forty-three use emerging characteristics of independence to increase their skills to cope with life's problems. The women became less defensive and showed greater self-esteem than they had previously demonstrated. These qualities coincided with greater commitments to work than they had reported in earlier years. The involvement in work did not replace their active roles as mothers but did begin to equal parenting as a responsibility.

19. Katie York and Oliver John, (1992), The four faces of Eve: A typological analysis of women's personality at midlife, *Journal of Personality and Social Psychology* 63(3):506–7. York and John looked at different factors but used the same women as Helson and Moane.

20. Ravenna Helson and Paul Wink, (1992), Personality change in women from the early 40s to the early 50s, *Psychology and Aging* 7(1):46–55. Ravenna Helson and Paul Wink's study found increased confidence and decisiveness as well as decreased feelings of dependence in women aged fifty-two. These women were mostly menopausal or postmenopausal, no longer had children living at home, rated their health fine and life satisfaction very favorably. Helson and Wink did not find that these changes were associated with menopause, empty nest, or involvement in caring for parents, so it was not a change in biology or caretaking that enabled the positive shifts to comfort, self-confidence, decision-making ability, flexible thinking, and tolerance of complex feelings and ideas.

Helson and Wink found women had an integration in personality characteristics that was not an increase in aggression or control, but rather a broader range of ways to think about life events; increased comfort with themselves; firmer commitments; and changes in roles and self-image. These researchers noted in a different study, with the same age group, that these women had time and energy to release in other directions and usually did so.

21. Valory Mitchell and Ravenna Helson, (1990), Women's prime of life: Is it the 50s? *Psychology of Women Quarterly* 14:451–70. Mitchell and Helson went to the heart of the matter with their question—do women have a prime? Cultural stereotypes suggest that women peak in late adolescence, perhaps because women are most attractive to men then. Also, late adolescence is a fertile time, and women's value has always been in maternity and sexual attractiveness. In 1983, from a large group of women, those who were in their early fifties (average age = 51) most often described their lives as "first-rate" as compared to the younger and older women in the sample. When the researchers went back to the same sample in 1989, the women who had reached their early fifties (average age = 52) also rated their quality of life as "high." In each group, whether they were fifty-one years old in 1983 or fifty-two

years old in 1989, the women showed confidence, security, involvement, and breadth of personality—the same kind of findings!

Mitchell and Helson also asked a series of questions that the women rated more true or less true than ten years before. The questions give us insight into why the women considered their lives first-rate. The seven items that more than three-fourths of the women rated as more true at age fifty-two were: being selective in what I do; a sense of being my own person, feeling established; more satisfied with what I have, less worried about what I won't get; focussed on reality; meeting the needs of the day and not worrying; feeling the importance of time's passing; and bringing both feeling and rationality into decisions. Thus the researchers concluded that most of the women felt that they had developed more control over their lives.

22. Nancy Andreasen, (1987), Creativity and mental illness: Prevalence rates in writers and their first-degree relatives, *American Journal of Psychiatry* 144:1288–92.

23. Ruth Richards, Dennis Kinney, Maria Benet, and Ann Merzel, (1988), Assessing everyday creativity: Characteristics of the Lifetime Creativity Scales and validation with three large samples, *Journal of Personality and Social Psychology* 54(3): 476–85.

24. Robert Weisberg, (1994), Genius and madness: A quasi-experimental test of the hypothesis that manic-depression increases creativity, *Psychological Science* 5(6): 361–67.

25. Arnold Ludwig, (1992a), Creative achievement and psychopathology: Comparison among professions, *American Journal of Psychotherapy* 46(3):330–56. Comparing people within the creative arts, theater people show more alcohol and drug use and more mania, anxiety, and suicide attempts, but not depression. Essay writers show adjustment problems before age forty, alcohol problems after forty, and depression throughout. Fiction writers show alcohol and drug use, depression, suicide attempts, and anxiety and adjustment problems before forty. Poets show similar use of alcohol and drugs, depression, and suicide attempts but display mania and psychoses before forty. Artists show more alcohol use, depression, anxiety, and adjustment problems throughout life. Musical performers show alcohol and drug use throughout and suicide before forty. Musical composers show alcohol problems before forty and depression throughout.

26. Donna Cangelosi and Charles E. Schaefer, (1992), Psychological needs underlying the creative process, *Psychological Reports* 71:321–22.

27. George Vaillant and Carolyn Vaillant, (1990), Determinants and consequences of creativity in a cohort of gifted women, *Psychology of Women Quarterly* 14: 607–16.

28. Bella Abzug with Mim Kelber, (1984), *Gender gap* (Boston: Houghton Mifflin).

29. Dean K. Simonton, (1992), Gender and genius in Japan: Feminine eminence in masculine culture, *Sex Roles* 27 (3,4):101–19.

30. Sharon Begley, (1993, June 28), The puzzle of genius, *Newsweek*, p. 50.

31. Virginia Woolf, (1929), *A room of one's own* (New York: Harcourt Brace Jovanovich), pp. 43–44. Jane Austen, one of the first women to describe women's experience, began her novels only two hundred years ago.

32. Ibid., p. 83. Woolf wrote, "A woman must have money and a room of her own if she is to write fiction" (p. 4), well aware that economic security was a myth

for most women and that women had none of the confidence that accompanies power and advantages.

33. Ibid., p. 11.
34. Ibid., pp. 92, 93–94.

❖   ❖   ❖

PART II
RECONNECT TO THE SELF

Even if we have avoided change before, midlife presents possibilities. Relinquishing old ways was just the beginning, maybe the most difficult. Next, we reconnect to ourselves.

Rollo May called creativity "the encounter of the intensively conscious human being with his or her world."[1] In art, we do not judge the greatness of a poem or painting by its exact likeness to clouds in the sky or a vase of flowers; we accept the artist's vision, the subjective world that resulted from her encounter with reality, the objective world. That can be our metaphor. We encounter life and its problems as honestly as possible, engage them completely, and use what we learn to construct a better life.

To encounter is to enter into a relationship. Carolyn, an occupational therapist who is also partially deaf, had never worked in the world of the hearing impaired. When she got a job working with deaf people, she "was confronted with an enormous amount to learn, but also had to face what it was doing to me . . . and I really began to think about what it meant to me to have grown up with an invisible handicap. People had no sense that I was perceiving the world differently, and basically I didn't know. I had no awareness of the impact that not hearing had on me." It opened up more than a career for Carolyn; as she put it, "it set me on my way."

To encounter is to make contact. It has nothing to do with winning or losing; it has to do with keeping the appointment, with being there. I do not refer to a physical presence only. As a child, I sat through geography lessons and never encountered the subject. As an adult, this still happens in other contexts. My use of the term "encounter" here refers to an emotional as well as a physical meeting, marked by receptivity to people, ideas, feelings, sights, and sounds outside of ourselves. Why? Because when we live exclusively within ourselves, there is not enough stimulation and excitement, not enough newness. Women are particularly good at being receptive to ideas and feelings from inside and outside, so we have a ready-made advantage.

With this advantage, we begin to think creatively as we bring ideas into our minds, take them apart, play with them, and toss them around until they become our own. The reconstruction is ours—how we put thoughts and feelings together, what we add or subtract, and how we turn it all around to reach new understandings. We have been slowed by trusting other people's judgments, relying on their vision. When will we trust our own vision?

When we encounter our world, we begin a passionate reforming of it by virtue of the encounter. Women have always lived that way; we mother that way, and we engage as wives, partners, and friends in that way. We may be uncomfortable with the notion that we are reforming the world, but what else can we call our devotion to raising children, to nurturing and maintaining relationships, to work, or to volunteering?

And in the process of changing the world, we change. It is not so easy to separate the managers from the managed, although we often tend to think of it as an either-or proposition; we do or are done to. We cannot change things or people without being changed ourselves; we change in the act of changing others.[2] It is at midlife that we can fully accept ourselves as reformers, recreators, or reshapers, because by then we have become more comfortable with the power required to enact reform. Power often connotes domination over others rather than collaboration. For those of us unsettled by power, we do well to remember that growth requires more than force; it demands a loving encounter with the world.

NOTES

1. Rollo May, (1975), *The courage to create* (New York: Norton), p. 56.

2. Frank Barron, (1963), Diffusion, integration, and enduring attention to the creative process, in R. W. White (Ed.), *The study of lives* (New York: Atherton Press), pp. 242–43.

❖ 5 ❖

"SHE MUST BRAID US ALL TOGETHER"
The Psychology of Women

Freud is the father of psychoanalysis. It had no mother.
  —Germaine Greer

If you are not wonder-working,
Who will have you?
  —Joyce Carol Oates

Some of us are becoming the men we wanted to marry.
  —Gloria Steinem

I attended a week-long workshop in Santa Fe, New Mexico. The presenters, all accomplished men and women, spoke to a filled auditorium each morning. At the end of the week, the most powerful reaction I had was not to the subject matter but to how very differently the men and women presented their work. Some of it was gender style: women laughed more than men, women apologized for requesting lighting or overhead equipment adjustments, and women were generally self-effacing, whereas the men made polite demands for equipment and service and seemed more comfortable telling a large audience what they thought. More disturbing were the differences in their presentation of material. The men presented their ideas and talked about how they had formulated these thoughts, how distinct their ideas were from all that had come before, and what unique contributions their work made. They stressed the individualistic qualities of their work. When women presented material, they cited their references, alluded to other writers, thinkers, and psychologists, and generally each woman presented herself as being one individual in a series, building on ideas that had come before. Women acknowledged the connectedness to other work. The differences made me angry, but I still am not sure at whom. It is a dilemma I, like many women, face all the time. I like the women's ways of relating; I identify with them and speak more like the women than the men, but I know that the men's style is valued more highly and that it certainly conveys more authority to a large audience. These different styles reflect underlying questions that apply to midlife women: what is uniquely my creation? What is created in connection with others?

The heart of women's psychology centers on the connections to others. We can no longer rely on antiquated theories that emphasize independence or individuation to the exclusion of relatedness. But the new emphasis on connection ignores the importance of the return to an individual self in the middle years.[1] All the research specifically examining the middle years finds that women do not lose their desire for affiliation, but they greatly increase their desire for autonomy. The balance of self and others is reworked throughout life, and in midlife, that balance is about changing relationships with children as they leave home, ending childbearing, coping with aging and ill parents, and rethinking new directions for our lives. We separate, individuate, and reconnect repeatedly. We separate from our children as they mature and rework new ways to relate and reconnect to them more appropriately as adults. We often distance from family, and even partners, since personal needs or dilemmas must be thought through before we are able to reconnect as somewhat changed women. We redo our relationships with work and community, and if we want to be creative, we make time to step back, to review, and to reconnect with ourselves in new ways. This juggling of our individual selves and our connections to others is a theme that runs throughout our lives. First, we look at the connectedness.

WOMEN'S CONNECTEDNESS TO OTHERS

Women live in relation to others, physically and emotionally. Traditional psychoanalytic theory emphasized separation, but this thinking never quite fit women's experience of their own lives. Much of what we have always valued, such as the centrality of relationships, was seen as pathological. Old theories held that disconnection, or disengagement of the mother-daughter bond was best for the daughter's development. A daughter demonstrated mental health by her ability to separate from her mother. This idea has undergone revision. In recent years, female development has been understood by looking at connectedness to others not as incomplete maturation but rather as a distinct line of development. Realizing the deficits in traditional theory, "a new model of development is needed to account for the centrality and continuity of relationships throughout women's lives."[2] Nancy Chodorow, Carol Gilligan, and others have furthered the understanding of relationships in the lives of girls and women. They propose that because girls see themselves as similar to their mothers, female identity develops in the context of that relationship. Boys see themselves, and are seen, as different from mother, and therefore find their identity in separateness. Masculinity is defined through separation and femininity through attachment.[3]

Bella Abzug, writing about the gap between men and women in politics, applies this same psychological theory to politics. She adopts the notion that men are guided by a sense of equality and justice and women are guided by an ethic of care, which includes concern with consequences, immediate situations, and personal relationships.[4] The "ethic of care" is Carol Gilligan's term for the concern women have for the feelings of others, even at times when care means that we exclude our own emotions or best interests.[5] Abzug noted that this ethic of care moves women to become involved with peace, environment, and the needs of others. These are the issues on which men and women consistently vote differently. Hillary Rodham Clinton was not put in charge of the Pentagon; she formulated health care. These values have been held by women for a long time. The difference now is that women are no longer ashamed of their values or consider them second-rate. At midlife, more than ever before, women feel greater confidence in their beliefs.

This ethic of care also explains problems that we experience. Women are comfortable with an ethic of care for *others*. Caring for ourselves and connection to ourselves has proved more difficult. Society, too, appreciates our care for others and admires that value, but does not have the same respect for women's self-care or self-interest. We have mirrored society's values, and fear that if we put ourselves into the picture it is the same thing as putting ourselves before others. We have always seen this as selfish and feared damage to precious relationships. Yet a complete ethic of care recognizes not only the legitimacy of others' needs but also the care of one's self, which allows for healthy self-interest, not selfishness: it allows us to also be acknowledged and included as worthy of concern!

HOW WE ARE FORMED BY OTHERS

Researchers and clinicians have been systematically exploring the idea that our experience of and our relationships with important persons in our lives influence the deepest aspects of our being. From birth throughout life, significant others have a hand in creating our character. They inspire our feelings of cohesion, well-being, and aliveness, basic elements in each of us. Important people shape our experiences of ourselves, of our lives, and of the world we live in, and in these ways, they also affect our relations with others.[6]

An interesting example of this was offered by redheaded Megan, forty-three, who was the youngest of six in a blue-collar, Irish Catholic family in Chicago. She had, from all outward appearances, separated in childhood; when the rest of her family all went off to work for the City of Chicago, she was the only one of the girls who went to college, had a good career, and traveled. Yet the image she held of her parents and older brothers and sisters for many years was that they knew everything and were bright and wonderful; she saw herself as little. That image, formed when she was a young child, when everyone else *was* bigger and wiser, had gone unchallenged into adulthood. The other half of her self-image, also developed in relation to her family, was that of self-sufficiency. The self-sufficiency grew because she had no one on whom she could depend. So she had an independent, tough, "I can do anything" quality mixed with the warm, earthy softness of the baby of the family who admires others. In her late thirties, she realized that she had been having trouble "growing up" and began a series of changes that resulted in the expansion of her self-sufficiency and toughness to include trust in others and increased softness. I attributed her change to marriage and happiness, but she explained that it had started some years before, beginning with her return to school and a new job.

As a child, Megan had developed in relation to her family and in accord with the vision of herself reflected in their eyes. As an adult, she continued to hold on to her childhood view of her family and their view of her. As she learned more about herself and about them, her views changed. She also had to face a clearer understanding of herself in relation to the members of her family.

The wish is so strong and the disappointment is so large that I didn't want to . . . come to terms with who they are. Well, the point was I was doing it all along; they were no help to me at all. Here, I had all these older brothers and sisters and they never helped me at all, and I realized that they didn't know how to. My sisters hadn't worked; there were no mentors, there were no teachers. . . . That's why I'm so much into this self-sufficient image of me as so strong; I had to be, growing up, and didn't realize that I could let my guard down now and depend on some people.

She learned as an adult that

there were people out there that could do what my family couldn't do. I didn't believe it. So it was actually doing that kind of separation, seeing that the whole world didn't fall apart, that made me realize that everything I'm doing feels good. Every change. . . . I like change, you know.

At first, the separation was sad. It was also a relief. . . . They didn't purposely mean to hurt me, they didn't know and couldn't understand anything else. That makes me angry. It makes me feel like I had abilities that weren't utilized. It all hit me in my thirties. Where am I going? What am I doing? I had no instructions from them.

In her new job, Megan met a woman a few years younger than herself with whom she became very friendly, and in that relationship, she had some startling insights. "Amy was a tremendous influence on my life; meeting her when I did. . . . She was so sweet and so kind, I used to think, 'This has got to be a put on; it's not real.' I wasn't used to it and I didn't trust it."

Megan's relationship with Amy challenged her belief that people were untrustworthy. "There was a real friendship and I could trust her and the idea of reciprocating—you can give me and I can give you—you don't always have to be always giving or taking. But still, I couldn't get that relationship with a man." As Megan realized that Amy's kindness and friendship were genuine, she learned the value of those qualities in close relationships.

Megan said that she needed to "accept all the parts of me—integrate them. They were so separated. I wouldn't even admit that I wanted to get married. It seemed like a weakness. I didn't understand it. You were supposed to go it alone. Toward my thirties, it wasn't as much fun. I did not want to be dependent on anyone. I always saw it as weak and I had to be self-sufficient and strong. I didn't realize you could be both self-sufficient and vulnerable."

The way Megan had taken care of herself in the past was with total self-sufficiency—never letting anyone get too close. Growing up, she had learned, "Don't depend on others." Although that thwarted her need for intimate relationships, her fear of dependency was stronger than her desire for closeness.

Recently she married for the first time. "My husband is so-o-o-o wonderful. He is a male Amy in the ability to be that giving and that caring. . . . I had realized that was what I wanted."

In Megan's story, we can see how parents and other important people influence the deepest aspects of ourselves. If they disappoint us, we expect disappointment from others, and it is possible that we will connect with people who will continue those patterns. If we had to be self-sufficient because parents could not help us in the ways we needed help, we will continue to be self-sufficient, although it may be in very distorted ways, such as taking care of an alcoholic husband. No parents are perfect. No childhood is perfect. Parent-child relationships are very human and therefore filled with stumbling and mistakes.

We each have been left a legacy. All of our childhoods leave something for us to work on in adulthood, but our basic sense of self begins early, and if those years were generally sound, we have a solid launching pad for our adult work. This self is a psychological structure that includes the sense of personal integration, meaning that we have an inner consistency; the belief that our life has meaning; and the experience that aspects of those people who are close to us can be a source of solace at times of distress.[7] This sense of self endures over time and continues to develop in the context of our present relationships.

Certainly each of us is born with a basic temperament, but here we see how people help create us simply through their interactions with us. Megan had grown up in family relationships that left her overly self-sufficient, with difficulty in tolerating some disappointments. Later relationships, like those she formed at school, at work with Amy, and with her therapist, helped her develop an ability to trust, to take responsibility for her actions, and to allow enough dependency to be close to others. These influences begin as people outside us and make their way inside as internal voices. As adult women, the voices inside will be the ones that inhibit us or grant us freedom to move on.

INTERNAL VOICES

From the viewpoint of traditional psychological theory, the self is built up from attributes of others represented in us, called "internalizations." Internalization describes a learning process. At the most basic level, learning might involve a baby sensing her mother's physical presence and figuring out how to anticipate her reappearance.[8] The infant senses the mother less as a real person with a real identity and more as a need-gratifying object (the term "object" in psychology refers to perceived characteristics, not always the entire person). Our children do not see our complexity any better than we knew our parents as complete individuals. Interactions between caretaker and child are repeated over and over again until the object is retained in the child's memory. At this point in a child's development, knowing that the perceived object will return to bring comfort helps the child accept needs like hunger or fear. She learns to tolerate and delay gratification of these needs. Later, the child uses her intellect to understand what the caretaker can and cannot provide at a specific time. The object is now inside and can be kept always. In this way, we learn to meet our own needs when the caretaker is not available. An example of this is when children sing to themselves at bedtime, just like mom usually does. Even in adulthood, we call on our "internal objects" to soothe us in times of distress, for example, by asking ourselves, "What would my mother, therapist, best friend, or big sister do now?" If we can keep gentle people with us—even when they are away from us or no longer alive—we are comforted. As we mature, we recognize more of the complexity of people and our relationships with them.

We internalize what we experience. Many, many years ago, my mother used to sing to me, so her voice is forever in my picture of her. If she had not, even if she had a terrific voice and sang to others, my personal picture of her would be different. This explains why there are so many distortions in our internalized objects.

Self psychology offers additional perspectives on objects and reminds us that what we call the "self" evolves from variations in our experience of others, particularly the early ones, in which we experience functions others perform for us as our doing, or extensions of ourselves, making them "self-objects." It is only later that we see their actions as separate from us. In adulthood, this leads to an understanding that real people provide essential functions and that we need relationships that contribute to our well-being and sustain us. The goal of individuation is not to free us totally from other people but rather to help us develop mature, interdependent relationships that are free of distortion and wishes and are capable of changing over time, depending on our needs.

Internalization is important for freeing creative activity in adulthood because the internal voices not only provide comfort and a measure of self-sufficiency but also allow us to take risks and try new adventures. If we do not have helpful, gentle internal voices, it is more difficult to soothe ourselves and to be vulnerable because the voices are harsh and critical. Instead of feeling loved, we feel persecuted. When we want to act, we feel uncertain; when we want to create, we feel untalented; when we try to listen to our own wishes, we feel frightened or insignificant. The process begun in childhood continues in adulthood, either through maintaining similar relationships with people or through holding on to the harsh internal voices from childhood.

Joan Riviere, an object relations theorist, noted how inextricably we are linked to each other:

We tend to think of any one individual in isolation; it is a convenient fiction. We may isolate him physically, as in the analytic room; in two minutes we find he has brought his world in with him, and that, even before he set eyes on the analyst, he had developed inside himself an elaborate relation with him. There is no such thing as a single human being, pure and simple, unmixed with other human beings. Each personality is a world in himself, a company of many. That self, that life of one's own, which is in fact so precious though casually taken for granted, is a composite structure which has been and is being formed and built up since the day of our birth out of countless never-ending influences and exchanges between ourselves and others. . . . [T]hese other persons are in fact therefore parts of ourselves, not indeed the whole of them but such parts or aspects of them as we had our relation with, and as have thus become parts of us. And we ourselves similarly have and have had effects and influences, intended or not, on all others who have had an emotional relation to us, have loved or hated us. We are members of one another.[9]

Internal voices are carried around inside us, and in that way, connect us to those people, good or bad, who have influenced us. When they are inside, we no longer require them outside because we know what they would say to us. For example, I can walk into any dress store and tell you what my mother would pick out for me, color and style, and how she would turn the dress over to check its hem and seams. I always have company while shopping. In these ways, the connections can either bind us or free us; they bind us when the voices are harsh and restrict freedom, and they free us when the voices are encouraging and we are able to take chances. In the shopping example, I still feel bound by color (never buy light green), style (keep it simple) and price (always check the sale racks). I am freed by a variety of circumstances (a new school year, good value, a celebration) that encourage me to make a purchase, and limited by others. This example is neutral, neither crippling nor enhancing. Let's first look at internalized voices that connect women to the past, but in crippling ways.

Years ago, I treated Susan, a dark-haired, dark-eyed, lovely Laura Ashley type. She was the youngest of five children, now in her mid-thirties and having a terrible time at work and in relationships. Her secretarial skills were excellent, so she had no trouble getting jobs, but she never stayed at a company long enough to get promoted. Whenever her supervisor asked her to do something or asked her neutrally if she had completed work, Susan heard it as criticism. When offered an independent project, Susan always refused because she was sure that she would fail. If her opinion was requested, she was literally speechless. Exactly the same thing happened in her relationships with men. She could not speak up because she was terrified of making mistakes, so she wound up with very domineering men who had all the opinions and made her feel increasingly small, until she left them or they tired of her. She wanted to be invisible. Once we identified this basic problem, she traced it back. A consistent memory was eating dinner in her parents' home, where she was ridiculed by her older brothers and sisters. Her sisters were talented; her brothers were noisy. They never understood how much they terrorized her. She became frightened of having an opinion of any kind and tried to become invisible. The problems from these relationships were compounded by Susan's terrible fear of talking to her mother because she seemed so overwhelmed by all these children to care for. Her mother was not evil or uncaring, but she had aspirations to status and was happier on committees or cleaning the pots and pans than getting into the emotional lives of her noisy children. The kids understood. One of Susan's saddest memories was an afternoon when she and her sister were riding together on a bike and both fell, collecting a good number of cuts. Her sister went into the house to be consoled by their mother, while Susan bandaged her own leg quietly in the upstairs bathroom. They knew that their mother could tolerate only one hurt child. Susan became an angry young woman. She had trouble believing anyone would care for her, so she simply tried to go along, and she became an expert at keeping quiet. In therapy, she had to relearn to think, to feel, and then to speak up again.

We overcome internal critical voices through good adult experiences that replace the harsh voices with gentler ones. Sometimes those experiences are with friends or husbands, and often they are with therapists. For Susan, the experience was therapy followed by a relationship with a gentle man whose manner comforted her. When I last heard from her, she was feeling safe, was able to listen to him and others, and could speak about her own experiences. This allowed her to take initiative in her work as well as make plans to marry.

As we develop in relation to others, we take in images of them and of ourselves. The image we each have of ourselves is influenced by others' reactions to us, their views of us, how we believed they felt about us, and all other aspects of our conscious and unconscious relationship with them. If they loved us, we experience ourselves as lovable. If they laughed at our jokes, we believe that we possess wit. If they didn't know us, it may be difficult to know ourselves or others. If they ignored us, we feel invisible. If they beat us, we feel the shame of an inherent badness.

Unlike Susan, Arlyne grew up in a home where children were enjoyed. Her experiences remind us of the internal voices that connect us to others in ways that allow creativity and freedom. Arlyne, an only child, is a forty-five-year-old business owner in Minneapolis who grew up in New York and left her large, extended family just to go to college in the Midwest, but met her husband as a freshman and stayed. Although they have had some rough times, she and her husband have developed a real partnership. This may soon extend to opening a business together. She recalled the support that she always counted on from both her mother and father.

My mother and father believed I was wonderful. I was just what they wanted. That has caused me plenty of problems about trying to deliver the goods, but, when all is said and done, no matter how bad things have gotten in my life, I hold on to their voices and actions that let me know I was good. It's hard to put the right words to it. It is probably the best thing they gave me. They did it differently: my mother was very soft and sympathetic; my father was quieter and could be gruff, but both of them managed to let me know that I was valuable.

She went on, "There were things that were limiting in the relationship I had with my mother, but the very nice thing was the sense that I was worth loving. I keep that with me. Sometimes when I have to do something or go someplace that frightens me, I wear her cameo pin. I started doing that after she died." Arlyne's self includes voices that provide self-esteem and confidence, two qualities that allow us freedom to act and to relate to others without losing ourselves. Thinking like this, individuation not only involves a distinctness and separateness, but also a particular way of being connected to others. All too often, we imagine that to individuate is to be alone. Instead, we can begin to think about new ways to be ourselves while we remain connected to others.

There are three crucial aspects of the mother-daughter relationship that foster development in the daughter. The first is the mother's continuing desire to be connected to her child. Society encourages more connection between mother and daughter than between mother and son or father and daughter. Attentiveness from her mother models interest in the well-being of others, teaching the daughter the value of listening to other people. I have often joked to my students that, as a psychologist, I do the same job my mother did sitting at the kitchen table, and not nearly as well.

In adulthood, we see the place of true attentiveness in love. Thinking long and hard about what had worked and failed in her marriage, one woman suggested, "I've come to think that really what love is, is a capacity to recognize another person, just recognize them. . . . And again, it has to do with the inside and then recognizing what's inside a person and also being recognized on the inside."

The second aspect of the mother-daughter relationship is mutual empowerment, where we are empowered by our closeness with our mothers because the closeness helped us feel competent in relating, so now we look for pleasure in emotional sharing. The ability to relate is valued among women, and the desire to continue to share emotions leads women to seek relationships throughout life.

The third aspect, the development of empathy, allows the daughter to keep a sense of herself and to appreciate her similarities to and differences from others.[10] Empathy includes both thinking and feeling as we attempt to understand another person's experience. A moderate delegate speaking in a National Public Radio interview during the 1992 Republican National Convention expressed this sense of empathy. Refusing to fight for a statement acknowledging pro-choice sentiments in the Republican platform, she explained, "It is difficult to hold out for what you want when you can see both sides of the issues."[11] This example also shows the way that understanding others can paralyze a woman and cause her to put aside her own interests. Interestingly, the ability to tune into the outside world is basic to creative talent: greater sensitivity to information received by our senses, unusual capacity for awareness of relations between various stimuli, and predisposition to a wider and deeper empathic ability than usual.[12]

Relating to others and understanding them becomes central to our power as women. Even in business, connectedness is noticeable and strong. Nancy talked about the artists who came into her craft store (which features work by women exclusively) with a great deal of respect.

Women are so happy to help other women. All they have to do is ask the questions. Many women have . . . asked us how we got started, how they come up with a wholesale price for their art, how to begin things . . . and it's empowering to them to get the answers and not feel intimidated, and it's important to me to give them information. . . . I'll never say to her, "I'm not going to pay you what you want." It's devaluing her work. Maybe we're just not the store that carries that particular item.

These are the connections. Now, let's turn to separation and individuation.

HOW DO WE BECOME SEPARATE INDIVIDUALS?

"She's needy. She's so-o-o-o dependent." We have all heard women disparaged in those terms. Maybe you have used "needy" or"dependent" to describe yourself. We shudder at the sound of these uncomplimentary terms. They imply that the woman in question cannot take care of herself. When was the last time you heard "needy" or "dependent" used to describe a man? They are terms used about women and against women. Our culture still reveres cowboys, independence, and rugged individualism above care and community. To admit to a need for others, to be less than self-sufficient, is ugly, inferior, and usually female.

What does it take for women to be separate, feel autonomous, be able to guide our own lives, and still have intimacy? To feel whole, we need both the connections and the individualism. The process of separation-individuation explains the dynamics involved in becoming a separate person. It begins in the earliest years of childhood and continues forever.

To be differentiated or individuated is to know oneself as distinct from others. To do this, we need a sense of safe, predictable personal and physical boundaries that separate us from other people.[13] Our skin is a primary boundary enveloping our bodies, just like our homes mark our physical space. We can imagine the horror if the boundaries of our bodies or our homes were violated. Individuation does not happen with one act—not as we go to school, get married, or leave town. Moves in the physical world are not necessarily moves in the psychological one. Individuation takes time and involves slowly becoming familiar with "me" and "not-me." As we mature, throughout life, we engage in the process of separating "me" from "not-me." Each time we do that, we become a more conscious individual. Midlife is an important time in this process. We become more complete and we develop a sense of our boundaries, where we begin and end and where others begin and end. We leave the undifferentiated jumble and claim a bit of ourselves. This gives us an identity.

Individuation is also becoming familiar with "you," which is different from "not-me." We learn to understand our mother as distinct from us, just as we learn to see ourselves as distinct from her. We learn that our mother has likes and dislikes and peculiar habits and ways of doing things, and this shows us that she too, is a separate person. Infants begin to realize this when their mother is late with the bottle or breast, when she does not pay attention or come quickly, or when she smells differently because she is wearing a new perfume. All these small differences gradually demonstrate the distinctness of us from her. If the separateness is too great—if she is depressed or has a long illness—it influences our view of the world. If the closeness goes on too relentlessly—if she limits our feelings or emerging abilities—that too influences our sense of being a complete individual.[14] Differentiation requires physiological growth, but physical maturity is not enough. A child develops through experiences of her mother's departure and return. An infant learns, through appropriately frustrating situations, that she has limited control of her mother. All these small, normal events teach us about being an individual.

Over the years, there have been significant changes in thinking about women's ability to individuate. Traditional theory held that an inability to separate completely inevitably made women less psychologically developed than men.[15] According to Freud, the best we could hope for was to idealize a man, depend on him, have his children, and then realize strength and creativity through them. Karen Horney, a follower of Freud, asserted a model of femininity that challenged Freud's idea. She insisted that women possessed positive qualities. She also went so far as to propose that "dread of women" exists because mothers are so powerful in all our lives. Mother's power is envied, and because the envy is intolerable, she is then devalued. This, Horney asserts, accounts for the devaluation of women.[16]

In traditional theory, independence was overvalued at the expense of interdependence. Neither men nor women ever attain complete independence from other people or from their environment. However, in healthy development, we grow from infantile dependency to mature interdependency. Conflicts concerning connections and separateness recur throughout our lives as we grapple with the balance between being with others and being alone. Is it okay to vacation alone? May I refuse lovemaking without feeling guilty? Without being punished? Do I have to sit here while you watch television? May I take time for myself? Ordinary situations bring the to-gether-alone questions up regularly. Midlife is another time to rethink connections and separateness. The balance that has worked in the prior years needs adjustment.

We individuate throughout life as we separate from others, as we separate from aspects of ourselves, as we relinquish old ways of relating to people, and as we develop new and better ways of being with others. We do it again as we mourn our losses, let go of the past, and enjoy our experience and knowledge. We know better than ever who we want to be and can find the courage to get closer to that ideal. We reestablish our personal boundaries of who we are and who we are close to. As long as we are willing to keep growing and creating our lives, we will need to shift our dependencies and our interdependencies. There is speculation that the ages between thirty and forty years old may be the normal time for women to fully individuate because it is then, having gained self-esteem, success, pleasure in mothering, having learned more about our own mothers, having achieved some distance from our childhoods, and having developed more realistic views of men, that we become more firmly our own persons.[17]

NO WOMAN IS AN ISLAND, EITHER

We are always linked to others, but the extremes become dangerous. True differentiation or individuation, then, is more than knowing self from other; it involves recognizing *two* selves, self and other. This awareness is not possible when we are either overwhelmed by our own needs or exclusively reacting to others.

Cynthia came into therapy overwhelmed by her own needs. She was in her late thirties, a talented watercolorist who could barely find the time or energy to paint because she was worried about painting, she was in an argument with her husband, or she needed more money, attention, or exercise. She was shocked when her husband said that he was thinking about leaving. Cyn needed so much, all the time, that she had lost sight of others as distinct individuals. People were tools to meet her own needs.

Flo was quite the opposite. She came into therapy briefly when she was fifty-two, and she was very bright, politically aware and overly devoted to her two daughters, who had both moved from the Midwest to the West Coast as quickly as they could. Flo was unemployed and could not think of work that she really wanted to do, although she was well read and educated. She had divorced her husband, the only action she could remember having initiated. Other than the divorce, Flo's life was one of reaction—first, to a very unstable mother who filled her with shame; next, to a husband whom she never loved; always, to her daughters, who were her life's work; and now, to a married man with whom she was having an affair. She knew he would never leave his wife, but she nevertheless hoped he would. Flo sadly reminded me of Marge Piercy's conclusion: a woman who makes love her career faces early retirement.[18]

Flo had come to therapy at her daughters' insistence, and they paid the bills. There, she waited for me to make it all okay. We talked for weeks about the problem of waiting and discussed alternatives, but there was nothing that Flo could act on, large or small. She waited for someone or something to react to.

When we recognize two selves, we can see the delicate balance—responsibility for others, but also for ourselves; care of others, but also for ourselves; and equal attention so we do not lose others, but certainly so we do not lose ourselves. (See Figure 7.) The potential problems in relationships can be located at the poles. Freud warned of the two extremes of relatedness: at one, the absorption with oneself to the exclusion of others, like Cynthia in her inability to see others except as extensions of herself; at the other, like Flo, a complete investment in others with a disappearance of the self, loss of energy, and no return of love.[19] Women can feel overwhelmed by their own needs and can be blind to others, but more often, we feel overwhelmed by the needs of others and cannot see ourselves clearly.

In Kate Chopin's beautiful, small book *The Awakening*, first published in 1899, the husband calls to his slowly awakening wife, who is sitting on the porch:

"You will take cold out there," he says irritably. "What folly is this? Why don't you come in?"

"It isn't cold; I have my shawl."

"The mosquitoes will devour you."

Balancing Self and Others

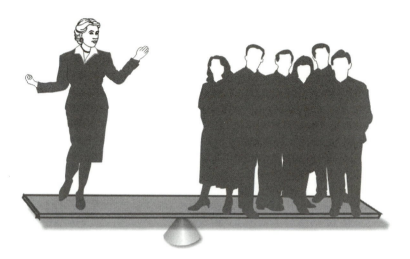

"There are no mosquitoes."

She heard him moving about the room; every sound indicated impatience and irritation. Another time she would have gone in at his request. She would, through habit, have yielded to his desire; not with any sense of submission or obedience to his compelling wishes, but unthinkingly, as we walk, move, sit, stand, go through the daily treadmill of life which has been portioned out to us.[20]

Later in the novel, the narrator notes about the husband, "It sometimes entered Mr. Pontelleier's mind to wonder if his wife were not growing a little unbalanced mentally. He could see plainly that she was not herself. That is, he could not see that she was becoming herself and daily casting aside that fictitious self which we assume like a garment with which to appear before the world."[21]

Intimate relationships change. Tolerance of both change and sameness is necessary for love relationships, particularly during periods of growth or upset. The women I spoke with were not immune to pain coming from their deepest connections with others. Some women were married, others were divorced. The married women valued the support of their husbands and were proud of their ability to maintain a cherished relationship. The women who were not married, and a few of the married ones, had faced problems that arise from relationships that were disconnected or not mutually empathic. Unsupportive relationships cause a decreased sense of vitality because of the sense of aloneness, a diminished ability to act because of the fear of further disconnection, less knowledge of yourself and others, a diminished sense of self-worth, and an increased likelihood that you will further isolate yourself to avoid more pain.[22] At worst, you begin to with-hold yourself from relationships in hopes of self-protection, but the result is a diminished sense of self and feelings of loss of an authentic self.

The women who had divorced were not sorry about their action and still believed in love relationships, but they certainly worried about the result of their divorce on their children. One said, "My marriage was so bad, but it took ages for me to stop kidding myself. I think that I was afraid that if I acknowledged the problems, I would have to do something about them, and I didn't know what to do. Sure enough, there really was no solution other than get out. Maybe if I had known all this years ago, I could have changed my marriage and kept it going. Who knows." Another resented the pity that came her way as a result of divorce. "The main thing I don't like about it, I realize, is a lot of people treat me as if this is a victim status. As if being a divorced person is 'oh dear, what happened?' I woke up. That's what happened." Another said, "I miss having a deeply loving relationship, but I didn't have that when I was married, so it really isn't the marriage I miss."

In a long-term study of emotional well-being of separated women and married women, it was found that marital separation led women to become more autonomous, a coping style that buffered stress. Therefore, separated women felt more confident and in control than their married counterparts. But these differences diminished over time as married women strengthened their abilities to cope within their families, using existing resources rather than finding new resources.[23]

Women, married and single, had become more comfortable with power. Earlier, they believed that everyone else had power and they simply reacted. At midlife, they recognized they also act and others react to them. "I had always thought I needed the institution more than it needed me, I needed Bill more than he needed me, I needed everything more than it needed me. . . . I realized that it wasn't necessarily the case." Women realized that their husbands and lovers were reacting to their changes. One admitted, "I've wondered my whole life about the impact I make. I know people make an impact on me; I'm just never sure that I make an impact on them. As I've gotten older, it has become somewhat easier to see. I think it has something to do with not wanting to see whatever power I possess." Another said that she had not felt accountable for relationships when she was younger because she always felt like the victim. As the women increasingly took more re-sponsibility for their lives, they became less afraid to exercise authority. As a result, the women also gained respect for the feelings that others may have had in response to them.

Whether they were in loving relationships or not, all the women I inter-viewed wanted an intimate partner. "I wanted to be able to mature and have a mature relationship. I wanted to be able to accomplish that. Ac-cepting that. Accepting intimacy on that level. That level of closeness. With no intimacy there is no real sharing as an adult, and I wanted that responsibility. That was being in charge of my life."

If we are healthy people who have internalized those whom we have loved, we are enriched by them always. Loss of love leads to distress, but it does not kill us, and loving allows us to survive.[24] Good attachment provides us strength forever, from childhood throughout life. The psychological work of mourning is more to remember than it is to forget. For most of my life, I have thought that the bad relationships I've endured were the ones that made the most impact on me. Now, in the middle years, I realize they provided more pain, not more influence. They were noisier, confusing relationships that lowered my confidence. The good relationships, even if they ended, had great power and still sustain me.

We have come full circle, then, from understanding what it means to be an individual to placing ourselves as separate in relation to others. It remains an eternal female struggle—to "be" and to "be with," to protect our personal boundaries and allow ourselves to be visited, not violated. As we mature, our bodies are visited by men in intercourse and by babies during pregnancies; we are the more "visited" gender. We have also become increasingly violated as rage is repeatedly directed toward women. Boundaries remind us that the difference between inside and outside should be respected. As women, we relate so much and are pulled in so many ways that it becomes all the more important to retain a sense of self that does not belong to mom, partner, kids, friends, or anybody. The women graduate students I teach always worry about combining the multiple demands in their lives, especially career and family. In ten years, not one male student raised that issue in class. Too much relating to others can result in feeling lost. I still remember the first time I stayed in a hotel alone after being married for ten years. I sat up in bed wondering very seriously if I wanted the light on or off. The idea of thinking only about myself was foreign; it had become easier to think about others. That night was more than twenty years ago, but it remains memorable because it scared me—not that there was danger from the outside, but because I realized that I had misplaced something inside.

Midlife changes some of life's demands. The children, if we had them, are older. We experience relationships differently, including increased concern with time available for ourselves and increased reluctance to continue poor relationships, which demand a great sacrifice of time and effort. We have more confidence: we are more willing to listen to ourselves and make our own mistakes, we can let go of some of the self-consciousness of young adulthood, and we do not want to play by other people's rules anymore. All this requires refinding whatever aspects of ourselves we have misplaced— our values, our wishes, and our dreams.

NOTES

Quote in chapter title is from Joyce Carol Oates, (1975), Wonders of the invisible world (poem), in *The fabulous beasts* (Baton Rouge: Louisiana State University Press), p. 7.

1. Linda Edelstein, (1995), Creative change as a result of midlife mourning (paper presented at the 103rd Annual Convention of the American Psychological Association, New York, New York).

2. Janet Surrey, (1985), Self-in-relation: A theory of women's development, Work in Progress, No. 13. (Wellesley, MA: Stone Center Working Paper Series). The Stone Center at Wellesley College in Massachusetts has produced some of the best ideas about self-in-relation theory as a way to conceptualize the development of women.

3. Nancy Chodorow, (1989), *Feminism and psychoanalytic theory* (New Haven: Yale University Press); Carol Gilligan, (1982), *In a different voice* (Cambridge, MA: Harvard University Press).

4. Bella Abzug with Mim Kelber, (1984), *Gender gap* (Boston: Houghton Mifflin), pp. 117–31.

5. Gilligan, *Different voice*.

6. Daniel Stern, (1985), *The interpersonal world of the infant* (New York: Basic Books). Using clinical experiments and observations, Daniel Stern has disproved one of Margaret Mahler's tenets that there is an undifferentiated bond between mother and infant, positing instead that infants have a core self from birth or before. Her 1968 book *On human symbiosis and the vicissitudes of individuation* (New York: International Universities Press) is important to this discussion because in it she describes the subphases of healthy child development, during which the infant begins to learn that she is a distinct person from her mother, that as mothers leave and return, children can also leave and return.

7. Ibid.

8. David Trosman, (1993), Differentiation through re-internalization: An exploration of internalized objects and the curative process in psychotherapy (Psy.D. diss., Chicago School of Professional Psychology).

9. Joan Riviere, (1955), The unconscious phantasy of an inner world reflected in examples from literature, in M. Klein, P. Heinmann, and R. E. Money-Kyrle (Eds.), *New directions in psychoanalysis* (New York: Basic Books), pp. 358–59.

10. Judith Jordan and Janet Surrey, (1986), The self-in-relation: Empathy and the mother-daughter relationship, in T. Bernay and D. Cantor (Eds.), *The psychology of today's woman* (New York: The Analytic Press), pp. 89–91.

11. National Public Radio interview, Chicago, August 19, 1992.

12. Phyllis Greenacre, (1957), The childhood of the artist, *Psychoanalytic Study of the Child* 12:47–72 (New York: International Universities Press).

13. Chodorow, *Feminism*, p. 102. Nancy Chodorow (1989) describes differentiation, or separation-individuation, as

coming to perceive a demarcation between the self and the object world, coming to perceive the subject/self as distinct, or separate from, the object/other. An essential early task of infantile development, it involves the development of ego boundaries (a sense of personal psychological division from the rest of the world), and of a body ego (a sense of the permanence of one's physical separateness and the predictable boundedness of one's own body, of a distinction between inside and outside).

Chodorow says, "Adequate separation, or differentiation, involves not merely perceiving the separateness, or otherness, of the other. It involves perceiving the person's subjectivity and selfhood as well. Differentiation, separation, and disruption of the narcissistic relation to reality are developed through learning that the mother is a separate being with separate interests and activities that do not always coincide with just what the infant wants at the time."

14. Ibid., p. 103.

15. Sigmund Freud, (1957a), Female sexuality, *Standard Edition* 21:223–46 (London: Hogarth Press). There have been significant changes in thinking about women's ability to separate over the years. The ideas proposed here are a shift away from traditional Freudian thinking. In Freudian terms, becoming autonomous for women meant to identify with the mother, and to accept their femininity, thereby resolving the Oedipus complex. A woman can then desire her father and men, without desiring to be men or to possess a penis, and will finally complete the detachment from her mother. The thinking was that we detach from mother, who has disappointed us for many reasons including not providing us with a penis, and we transfer affection to father and men. Then, we idealize men and remain dependent upon the man's strength, support, achievement, and power in a way that inhibits our own sources of assertiveness and creative expression. This was considered as good as autonomy ever got for women. Not surprisingly, penis envy was one of the concepts that was tossed out in feminist thinking. The Freudians never quite believed that women could separate because the thinking was inextricably linked to anatomy—lack of penis. We no longer consider this normal, although it was considered healthy feminine development at one time.

Freudian theory went so far as to say that as women, we were innately less developed because of our incomplete separation. Independence was valued as the primary goal of youth and adolescence. Interdependence was not discussed.

16. Karen Horney, (1967), *Feminine psychology* (New York: Norton).

17. Doryann Lebe, (1982), Individuation of women, *Psychoanalytic Review* 69: 63.

18. Marge Piercy, (1980), Shadows of the burning, in *The moon is always female* (New York: Knopf).

19. Freud, Female sexuality.

20. Kate Chopin, (1972), *The awakening* (New York: Avon Books), p. 52. Originally published 1899.

21. Ibid., p. 96.

22. Jean Baker Miller and Irene Stiver, (1991), A relational reframing of therapy, Work in Progress, No. 52 (Wellesley, MA: Stone Center Working Paper Series), p. 2.

23. Geoffrey Nelson, (1994), Emotional well-being of separated and married women: Long-term follow-up study, *American Journal of Orthopsychiatry* 64(1): 150–60.

24. George Vaillant, (1985), Loss as a metaphor for attachment, *The American Journal of Psychoanalysis* 45(1):59.

"I Am Her Only Novel"
Relationships with Parents and Their Dreams for Us

If we tried to sink the past beneath our feet, be sure the future would not stand on it.
—Elizabeth Barrett Browning

You will do foolish things, but do them with enthusiasm.
—Colette's advice to her daughter

I have made my world and it is a much better world than I ever saw outside.
—Louise Nevelson

As we age and our parents age, we gain a new awareness of our similarities to and differences from them. We see more clearly how they shaped us, good and bad. We see, too, how we, often unknowingly, carried their unfulfilled dreams.

One of the most complex changes in the middle years involves the shift in responsibilities from our parents and their generation to us and our generation. Our parents, having had a lifetime before we arrived, will forever be the "real grown-ups" somewhere in our minds. Their aging and death profoundly affect us, whether we are twenty or forty, whether the relationship has been nourishing or tortured. As they age or fail, we begin to assume responsibility for their care. For those of us who could never count on our parents, to care for them is depleting. For those of us who have been close to our parents, we have the chance to return old favors, but we lose parents as a source of support. We become their support. We are often forced to make decisions about their care, and perhaps agonize over decisions about living arrangements or life support techniques. We must think about the type of relationship we want with them, and in thinking about the changes needed to create that relationship, we must look at ourselves and decide if there are other changes we need that may be long overdue in our lives.

Eventually we must own the dreams our parents had for us as belonging to us or give them up if they are not dreams we can accept and live. Knowing all this, our childhoods end and we become the generation in charge.

CARING FOR AGING PARENTS: THE SHIFT IN SUPPORT

Although many women anticipate caring for aging parents, it is with mixed emotions. Some of us welcome the opportunity to repay old kindnesses. Others of us dread increased involvement with difficult parents. It is hard to care for a parent who has not cared for you. Either way, during the middle years, most of us have to say good-by to our parents as parents-in-charge. Unfortunately, caring for parents is not like caring for children, because it happens in the context of physical failures rather than in anticipation of growth and development.[1] The beauty and rewards of mothering are in the healthy development of our children. The work pays off. The worry, the physical exhaustion, the expense of time, energy, and money is worth it when the children turn out well. All the work and worry in the world cannot save a dying parent or reverse their decline. Cassie's father has Alzheimer's disease, and her mother has assumed total care for him. Cassie tries to help, but the disease feels endless to her and there are days when she simply wants to get on with her own life. Marilyn's widowed mother-in-law is showing signs of memory deterioration from years of alcohol abuse. She lives far away, so her daily care will not fall to Marilyn and her husband, but they worry about her safety and ability to take care of herself. Our help can make our parents more comfortable. We can be proud and satisfied to provide care, but the physical failures cannot be undone, so we fight the feelings of resentment when we try too hard and we receive no response, and we suffer with pangs of selfishness when we do not try hard enough. As adult daughters, we struggle with guilt over what we can do to help and what is impossible, with our desire to force our parents to live differently, make friends, visit doctors, or a hundred other ways we believe they could enrich their lives and be less isolated. We struggle to accept our own limitations and our fears.

Dorit, a friend and fellow psychologist, noted the many close connections that remain from relationships begun years ago. Although she believes that the midfifties is a time of personal growth and expansiveness for her, she is aware that "I'm tremendously loyal. I maintain old connections [and] it has a lot of love in it. . . . People that I love are sick, so there is no freedom to live my own life." Time is precious to Dorit. She spent many years raising children. Now the children are launched but she sees older friends becoming ill, anticipates the day when her mother's health will fail, and says, "There is no way I would pull away from my mother." When one friend became ill, it brought home the conflict: "An old friend calls, but her life is shrinking and mine is expanding."

For those of us who were lucky and received support and comfort from our parents, we lose that as they age. They were the people who always believed in us. For years after my mother died, I carried around this terrible sensation that if I ever turned around to look for help, no one would be there. I realized how many times I had counted on my parents to be there—not to do anything, not to even be anything, for I was far too independent for that; just to be. A heartwarming moment at my mother's funeral occurred when my older daughter Jenny, then twelve, wrote a poem that included a reference to no longer being able to hear the sound of her grandmother's voice—the small personal moments bring it home.

How They Shaped Us

The older generation has meanings for us other than simply as the people who raised us and for whom we will now care. We learned who and what women were all about from those people, especially the women. We watched them—mothers, aunts, grandmothers—and thought about who we wanted to become and who we did not want to become. Whether we like it or not, they are the yardsticks by which we measure our lives. I have had innumerable women come into therapy saying, "I see myself doing things just like my mother, and I swore I wouldn't." Last week, a normally reticent fifty-three-year-old woman threw herself into a chair and groaned, "I looked in the mirror and saw my mother—I'd rather see Richard Nixon!" Our reactions are strong if we fail women relatives, become them, or pass them by. We have learned a great deal from the women in our lives.

Margaret, raising two grade school children, talked about the important women in her family:

I was very close to one of my grandmothers who died when I was about twenty-six. I grieved for her when she died but I just thought, that's life and the old are going to die. But with children in my life, I started to think about her a lot more and think how I wish she had met these children, how delighted she would have been with them. In a funny way, she came back into my life as a real presence. It was realizing how a lot of her life had been deeply unhappy that made me realize that I didn't want the second half of my life to be like the second half of her life. So it's connected to a vision that I have of her. But it's not because she died then, but it was because of the way she lived, and thinking about it as I approached her age when her life started to turn bad. . . . A very sad life, always serving other people and always doing the best for others, and forty years of her life spent with happiness being just a glimpse now and then.

In remembering her grandmother, Margaret concentrated on the later years of her grandmother's life and compared them to her own future. Margaret knew that she did not want to duplicate that unhappiness. These memories drove her to face the unhappiness in her life and make adjustments in order to change the future she foresaw. She wanted to model her life on other attributes that were also in the women in her family.

I've always been energetic. And, well, I come from a line of matriarchs. . . . For generations the women in my life have all been tough cookies, and they've all been workers. My grandmother ran away from home because they wouldn't let her go to the college she wanted. My great grand mother ran away from Germany because she didn't like the idea of her young husband being in the Franco-Prussian wars. Women who move; who kept going.

There was a lot of sexism in my family when I was growing up. My brother's going to college was much more important than my going to college. . . . All of those things were of high value and those were not particularly valued for me. "Tom, get A's; you've got to get A's or you won't get into graduate school." That was the talk, but, in fact, . . . my mother always worked. So the model I had was of women who worked or women who did what women could.

Margaret's story about the women is typical of her generation—a lineage filled with women who worked if they needed to, tried to do things they wanted to, and were trapped by severe limitations on all sides.

In her autobiography, Eleanor Roosevelt also recalled her grandmother's influence.

She was the kind of woman who needed a man's protection. Her willingness to be subservient to her children isolated her, and it might have been far better, for her boys at least, had she insisted on bringing more discipline into their lives simply by having a life of her own. My grandmother's life had considerable effect on me, for even when I was young, I was determined that I would never be dependent on my children by allowing all my interests to center in them. . . . I am sure that my grandmother's life has been a great factor in determining some of my reactions to life.[2]

Melanie, on the other hand, felt that her early years were shaped entirely by

being the favorite child of my father. My father was the person who said, "You can do anything." My father was a Greek immigrant who jumped ship and told me every day, "You can be a doctor; you can be a lawyer." I never had to resort to wily ways to get what I wanted. We treated each other like business partners. He would consult with me. When I was nine years old, he told me this business problem and I said, "Dad, you're going to have to fire Charlie because he is stealing from you." He went and fired Charlie. Then you read *The Drama of the Gifted Child*, and you see the craziness that type of childhood brings on you because you think that you have all this power.[3] You know you are not smart enough to be giving your father advice, and you feel guilty because, "Why aren't you talking to Mom, she's thirty and I'm only nine." I never understood. I thought I was the luckiest person in the world to have a father who laid out all that stuff on me. I loved him dearly and he thought I was wonderful.

But when my father died, my mother wanted to kill herself, didn't care about us; she didn't want to live. A year later, when I was hit by a car and landed in the hospital with a brain concussion and a spine concussion, my mother sort of went,

"Oh gee, something could happen and it might even be worse than what just happened."

Her mother did recover and now they are very close. "I liked the way she was with me. She was a giving, giving person and I tried to be a giver like she is, to my kids. There wasn't much about my mother that I didn't want to be like, [but] I think I was patterning myself after my father. He was my soul mate. He was the one."

Women at midlife may be particularly open to a recognition of connections with previous generations as they experience the growing maturity of their own children and gain new perspectives on their parents' experience.

Their Dreams for Us

It did not surprise me that most of the women knew, with certainty, the content of their parents' dreams, especially their mothers'. Each of our mothers was different and so were their dreams for us. It is good that we know the dream, because knowing is the first step to making a real choice about whether or not we want any part of it.

Belinda, a writer, quickly answered when I asked about her mother's dream.

Is it possible to think of people as having two sets of expectations? My mother was, and is, a firm traditionalist, although she always worked. If you ever asked her what her life was about, it was always in the home. She had her own business, but she didn't value herself for that. She's a fabulous decorator, fabulous cook, and gave great parties, and that's where she just seemed to really relish her life. And business was business. She never acted burdened by it; . . . that's what you do, you work. I don't know if she had to work for money. . . . So my mother wanted me to be a real traditional woman, and still does. She's in her seventies, and she gets dismayed that I don't do dinner parties. She gives me crystal and crystal . . . just gorgeous. . . . If she had to write down, what do you think is most important to you, she would have said home life, or something like that.

Belinda was divorced, and that did not fit with her mother's dream.

My mother thinks that the definition of a woman is in a family, and if she's not married anymore, then she's shaky, even though my main definition is that I've got a good career; I've got lots of perks. She likes that, but she's worried. But [both my parents] are very proud of my work. They like me being out in the world. They've never read anything I've written. I mean, they just keep copies of it on the shelves and stuff, but they don't read it. But that's okay. They can see my name.

The dream Emma's mother had was less benign and remains a source of friction in their relationship. Emma, married, forty-three, now working in public relations, had lived most of her mother's dream for eight years—money, status, membership in a country club, and charity work. Then, when her husband's alcoholism sent him into the hospital, the dream unraveled and she found out that all the money was gone. It was going to be up to her to pay the bills. "We had lived a pretty extravagant life. I thought it was available." Emma had to make adjustments very quickly. The losses certainly shattered Emma's dream, but it also angered and confused her parents.

I was totally influenced by them before the first hospitalization, and somewhat after. They believe in marriage; they wouldn't have taken the easy road out of marriage. That was positive. They gave me the strength to believe in myself, but they don't understand the illness; they don't like what Gene has done to me. My mother thought I could be what she always wanted to be, which was a Pacific Heights volunteering grande dame. Now that is less important to her *for me*, but still important to her *for her*. It's more important to have the correct clothes than to pay attention to what someone is telling you. My father's family is quite prominent; hers was not. She had to put this persona on which was not comfortable for her initially, [but she adapted] hook, line, and sinker.

Emma added with dripping sarcasm, "She wasn't keen on our eviction from the apartment."

Emma's parents were disappointed in the way her life was turning out. They "could not deal with it. They provided no comfort, couldn't talk about it. I had to ask for financial help. They never offered because they felt it was my husband's financial mess." Her parents would have preferred that she leave Gene and return to their home, but this is where Emma took over her own life. "I think I began to see the other possibilities. I gained a perspective that is healthier. I have acquaintances that are into acquiring physical goods. How many shoes do you need? Why did I think that was important?"

Emma remained with her husband and made it work, and in the process, redefined her own dream, which now includes work, attention to relationships, having a voice in financial matters, and, very important, being a good mother. "I'm a better mother to my daughter. She can make her own decisions, her own mistakes. I give her that freedom. I don't overcontrol her like I believe my mother overcontrolled me. I learned."

Studies that followed educated women from college graduation in the sixties found that many women developed a career identity in addition to their commitment to domestic roles. Their commitment to careers reflected a change in feminine roles and a shift away from the role choices of their own mothers and toward the role choices of their fathers. Good relationships with parents predicted higher self-esteem at midlife than poor parental relationships. Similar values was also correlated to positive parental relationships, even when daughters had chosen different roles from their mothers.[4] An earlier study found similar results: women activists who believed that their values were in sync with their parents' values considered themselves more assertive and confident than women who experienced disharmony with parental values.[5] Continuity with parents helped self-esteem. However, only positive relationships with mothers predicted subsequent emotional well-being, probably because mothers continue to play a more active role in their daughters' emotional lives, thereby contributing to positive support that helps well-being.

BECOMING THE GENERATION IN CHARGE

In the middle years, each woman's relationship with her parents must change. Even if they have died, we move as we age, not into their shoes, but into well-fitting shoes of our own. They have shaped us, but in our middle years, we take responsibility for the rest of our lives, and for the lives of generations to come.

In the arrogance of our teens and twenties, we figured that when we grew up and reached the plateau of adulthood, we would magically know what we were doing. That has turned out to be untrue, and ignorance seems to go on forever, but we have not arrived empty-handed. The good news is that we are in charge; the bad news is the same.

There is a parable about old wise women who are asked by worried towns-people, "Does it make sense that humans have evolved on the earth?" The women go away, ponder the question, and return with the answer, "It does not make a lot of sense that we are here, but we are, so let's make it count."

One aspect of becoming the generation in charge is that we can reclaim the essential dream we had for ourselves. There is no way to begin all over again, but buried in other people's expectations for us and the diverse paths we have already walked, there are essential elements of dreams that remain and can be reclaimed. The decisions that we felt forced into or went into blindly, or that were imposed on us by work or family roles, may have limited us, but old motivations can be brought into awareness. Conscious-ness is the first step in modification. Some women, I have realized, are more comfortable old than young and find greater freedom with age.

The heart of old dreams can be brought forward in adult form. We can sort through our parents' and grandparents' dreams for us and see if they match our dreams for ourselves. It is in these actions that we begin to live life more authentically.

We also see that creative maturity is in the work and the actions rather than in the outcomes or the goal. Adult creativity must be in the relationship with ourselves and with others. Integrity exists when we behave according to the values that give meaning to our lives. Years ago, when I worked with people who suffered great losses, I realized that we get no guarantees of longevity or permanence in any creation, whether it is children or work or artistic productions. In seeing the pain that follows great loss, I also learned

Review and Decide

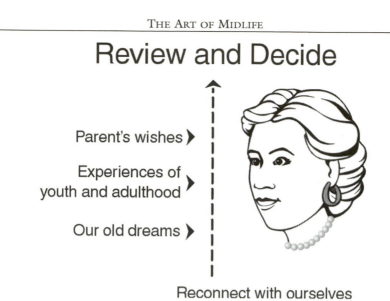

Parent's wishes ❯

Experiences of
youth and adulthood ❯

Our old dreams ❯

Reconnect with ourselves

that no one gets a "do over" as I insisted on years ago when a game call was questionable. We are shaped by all that happens to us, but, as suggested in Figure 8, we can use all of our experience to make the rest of our lives richer, free,r and more genuinely our own.

NOTES

Quote in chapter title is from Marge Piercy, (1980), My mother's novel (poem), in *The moon is always female* (New York: Knopf), p. 43.

1. John Oldham, (1989), The third individuation: Middle-aged children and their parents, in J. Oldham and R. Liebert (Eds.), *The middle years: New psychoanalytic perspectives* (New Haven: Yale University Press), pp. 93–94.

2. Eleanor Roosevelt, (1937), *This is my story* (New York: Harper & Brothers), pp. 300–301.

3. This is a reference to Swiss psychoanalyst Alice Miller's (1981) *The Drama of the Gifted Child.*

4. Wendy Welsh and Abigail Stewart, (1995), Relationships between women and their parents: Implications for midlife well-being, *Psychology and Aging* 10(2):181–90.

5. Jeanne Block, (1972), Generational continuity and discontinuity in the understanding of societal rejection, *Journal of Personality and Social Psychology* 22:333–45.

❖ 7 ❖

"THERE'S STILL SO MUCH I'D LIKE TO SEE"
How We Are Formed by Social Forces

It occurred to me when I was 13 and wearing white gloves and Mary Janes and going to dancing school, that no one should have to dance backward all their lives.
   —Jill Ruckelhaus

I became a feminist as an alternative to becoming a masochist.
   —Sally Kempton

Once in a cabinet we had to deal with the fact that there had been an outbreak of assaults on women at night. One minister . . . suggested a curfew: women should stay home after dark. I said, "But it's the men who are attacking the women. If there's to be a curfew, let the men stay at home, not the women."
   —Golda Meir

Like their personal lives, women's history is fragmented, interrupted; a shadow history of human beings whose existence has been shaped by the efforts and the demands of others.
   —Elizabeth Janeway

The women interviewed were shaped by more than temperament, parents, and relationships with others. They are women brought up in a country dramatically transformed after World War II by civil rights, Vietnam, and the feminist movement. National movements and events such as these occur in each generation and have great impact. Being part of one generation rather than another has profound results. We struggled to blend freer possibilities with our parents' conventional teachings and spent our first forty years making room in our identities for the conflicting images of Donna Reed, Marilyn Monroe, Hillary Rodham Clinton, and even Madonna. Womanhood has become increasingly complicated with an ever-changing relationship to our environment as we absorbed our culture, experienced national and world events, and responded to society's expectations, if not always immediately or consciously. Didn't we wear bell-bottoms?

More important than fashion influences are the subtle messages we received that said we could not do things, like enroll in shop classes at school, succeed in math, manage money, or train for certain jobs. We were often guided into "more appropriate" directions for "girls." When I was sixteen, I took the civil service examination to get a summer job at the local post office in the New Jersey town where I grew up. A man called afterward and told me that I had scored the highest, so they had to offer me the job but I could not take it because it was for a boy. I agreed and did not think that it was strange until years later. Neither did my parents. That kind of response was accepted as normal, and was intended to fit young ladies into society, not to harm us or make us feel limited or useless. Looking back, it is shocking to see how many limits there were and how many of the roles that we were encouraged to assume taught us to help others and nurture lives other than our own. As adult women, most of us still feel guilty if we stop being helpful.

Psychological studies of adult personality development have been criticized for ignoring conditions in the social world and the impact of these conditions on particular cohorts. Psychologists tend to look at people as individuals or within families, leaving the analysis of larger influences to sociologists and historians, although social forces have had a major impact in creating us as psychological beings. The timing of our births had a decided effect on our individual lives and spirits and gave us membership in the post–World War II generation, having grown up with civil rights, Vietnam, and the feminist movement. We never fit the blueprint for men's lives, but now we do not fit the old models for women's lives either. These forces create an environment that affects the way we feel about ourselves and our lives, affects others' feelings about us, influences our relationships with family and friends, informs our choices or lack of choices about work, and tells us to what extent we have value as members of society. What do these forces mean for creative living at midlife?

MEMBERSHIP IN THE POST–WORLD WAR II GENERATION

Our parents and grandparents lived through the Depression and World War II. Many of our parents emigrated from other countries or were the first generation born in this country. We are the children of sacrifice. Wherever they came from and no matter how long they had been American, the Depression and World War II left fear. These attitudes and anxieties are passed along within families, often unspoken. Whatever business has been left unfinished by one generation seems to appear, in some form, in the next. Carl Jung, the Swiss psychologist, noted, "All the life which the parents could have lived, but of which they thwarted themselves for artificial motives, is passed on to the children in substitute form."[1]

Certainly we each begin with a basic temperament and grow up in families that provide nourishment that will feed or poison our emerging spirits. But we also develop in relation to our social environments, although we each respond differently to events. In our generation, there was no shortage of events to make an impact.

Families changed dramatically after World War II. To understand the change, we have to take a look at the role of women in World War II. During the war, married women worked outside the home, which in itself was unusual, but they also took jobs in factories and other types of work that were previously unheard of for middle-class women. And they loved it! A Women's Bureau survey found that four out of five working women wished to stay in the labor force after the war. But as soldiers returned, women were laid off. The end of the war understandably marked a push for family "normalcy," which meant a return to life as it was before the war. The layoffs were fueled by the desire to have men back in jobs, the fear of an economic recession, and the persistent hostility to equality for women in the workforce.

In the year 1947, nearly one out of every two babies born was the first child in its family. We enjoyed economic good fortune as children. Those were also years of buying homes and moving to the suburbs, places that had never before existed. In spite of babies, layoffs, and homes miles away from the cities, women, including married women, persisted in their desire to work. They eventually found jobs—more menial and less remunerative than the jobs they held during the war. Even when women secured the same jobs as men, they were paid far less money. In *The Paradox of Change: American Women in the Twentieth Century*, history professor William Chafe wrote:

The absence of greater progress in the areas of equal pay, job segregation, community services, and recognition of women leaders raised profound doubts about the war's permanent impact on underlying attitudes toward woman's place. There could be little question that the economic role of women had expanded during the fighting. The sharp increase in employment of married and middle-aged women provided just one measure of the extent to which the war had changed women's lives. On the other hand, the hiring of millions of women did not itself signify that women had gained the right to be treated as equals with men in the job market. Economic equality could be achieved only through a substantial revision of social values and a lasting modification in the nature of male-female relationships.[2]

By 1952, ten million wives—our mothers—held jobs, more than at the peak of World War II. But attitudes did not seem to match the behaviors. A husband who previously might have opposed his wife's working now rationalized her job on the basis of economic inflation and family needs that would be satisfied by her additional income. At the time, women gave similar reasons for working; 84 percent cited "economic need" or the desire to "help the family" as the reason for working. "Thus, women workers themselves were, apparently, not seeking to challenge existing sexual roles. Instead, they were fulfilling the sanctioned function of 'helpmate' in a new way."[3] At least, that is what they were saying.

Forty years later, we see similar findings. Research has demonstrated that women's employment outside the home can have positive physical and mental effects on the wives; it is still not certain whether husbands experience positive effects when their wives work. More recently, researchers from the University of Michigan asked questions similar to those asked after World War II of married men who had grown up in a different climate. There were three groups of husbands—those with career-pursuing wives, those with working but not career-pursuing wives, and those with homemaker wives. Results showed that husbands of working women (who worked to help the family) and husbands of career women (who worked also for personal gratification) reported greater participation in housework than husbands of homemakers. Husbands of career wives reported the lowest depression but greater anxiety. This may be because career women may present too strong a challenge to husbands and the men assume additional household responsibilities. Homemakers' husbands fare the worst in terms of well-being, because they bear the sole burden of financial support. Husbands of wage earners seem to get the most benefits. They have financial help and may justify their wives' work as helping the family rather than as a means of personal gratification for their wives.[4]

Even years ago, for many women motivations were more complex, and economic need was a convenient justification. "Nevertheless what remained most significant was the *impression* that women sought to work out of necessity" rather than from personal desire or for fulfillment.[5] Helping others made work acceptable, but self-esteem, enjoyment, power or ambition made employment unacceptable.

The postwar debate on a woman's place continued. The most basic argument said that the temperament and anatomy differences between women and men determined that a woman's place was in the home. The argument, in its most rudimentary form, went as follows: a woman's psychic life was shaped by biology. Whether biology was seen as negative, the lack of a penis, or positive, the ability to bear children, the result of the biological differences meant that "normal femininity" required women to repress aggressive strivings or self-interest and to find, instead, success through a husband and the creation of a good home for him and the children.

Divorce rates exploded in the 1960s. That phenomenon killed whatever was left of the nineteenth-century sex-role system. The percentage of married women who worked went from 15 percent in 1950 to more than 50 percent in the 1980s. Our mothers—the conventional ones we still think of as Harriet Nelson incarnate—were the ones who went back to work. As the children who grew up after World War II, we carry our parents' changes on our collective psyches.

The decade of the 1960s brought about many profound changes. During the early years, we were enchanted by John Kennedy and his hopeful, youthful leadership. We paid more attention to his charm than to the Cuban missile crisis and the threats of war that had us standing in school corridors during innumerable air raid drills. The assassination of President Kennedy left a void in leadership, and briefly the generation gap disappeared as grief was shared by the nation.

There was a radical shift in the midsixties. Politics changed. Race has always constituted a central theme of American history, and the nation became alert to the inequalities of discrimination. We witnessed the passage of the Civil Rights Act of 1964, followed by murders and racial incidents from Selma to Watts. No protest movement occurs in a vacuum, and it is unlikely that feminism could have gained the energy it did during the 1960s without being fueled by the civil rights movement. The struggle to end racial discrimination opened women's eyes to a heightened consciousness about gender discrimination. The 1964 Civil Rights Act prohibited employment discrimination based on sex as well as race, although the inclusion of sexual discrimination had been made in an effort to squash the bill, not to help women. Betty Friedan's book *The Feminine Mystique*, published in 1963, although very middle-class in its attitude, marked the beginning of a feminist surge not felt since the suffragette movement to gain economic and social equality for women.[6]

Later in the decade, there was Vietnam. If ever there was a coming-of-age, it was through this war. Political analysts say that no post–World War II event left as great a scar on the collective psyche as Vietnam. "Viet Nam tore away any remaining myths or innocence the generation possessed about war and warriors," wrote Myra MacPherson of the *Washington Post.*[7] The average age of the soldier in Vietnam was eighteen to nineteen years old, as compared to thirty years old in World War II. As the country music song describes, young men went to war as their "class trip," and the divisiveness would stain decades to follow. Although not everyone experienced the same events in the same way, we did share Vietnam, whether we protested against or supported the war. We struggled with the morality of the war throughout adolescence and young adulthood and were still impressionable enough to be stunned by Watergate and the resignation of President Richard Nixon.

These political and social events marked our generations in personal ways beyond the obvious. There were questions of employment and careers; there was an increasing disenchantment with authority and politics accompanied by a sense of disconnection from the mainstream; and there was divorce. Feminism, even if you never read the books or joined a protest, gave rise to issues that reached into everyone's hearts. Throughout the 1970s, there were heated debates, not only with regard to equal employment, but in all sectors of life, including child care, "open marriages," abortion, household responsibilities, and sexual behavior. These were not mere intellectual dorm debates. Values about dating, loving, and marriage were all chaotic. Half of us were married guiltily in white in traditional houses of worship, and the rest were reciting Gibran prose as vows under the trees. Men and women faced changes in all aspects of daily life. As baby boomers, we are more educated than any generations in history; we married later than our mothers, so more of us worked; we have had smaller families; more of us are single parents; more of us have experienced divorce; and more of us are working, however young our children are. We have known that we must plan for living longer, statistically until eighty years of age, and often alone. We still make less money than men; and although median incomes have gone up, it is not as fast as inflation has risen, so our money does not stretch as far as our parents' paychecks.

Political scientist Paul Light comments on the different perceptions of men and women: "Many baby-boom women continue to believe that there are two American economies—one for men which is supported by aggressive federal policies, and another for women supported by no one but themselves."[8]

We have lived with decades of contradiction. Although the world had been turned upside down by the radical changes that had ensued in employment, sexuality, divorce, and family relationships, the persistence of inequality by gender and race made it seem as though little had been gained. Our lives are still filled with incongruity. No wonder we lost our beliefs in traditional institutions; they became irrelevant to our real lives. Our generations are tolerant of more social diversity but are disillusioned with political leaders and marks of status. Many of us have rejected traditional social roles in the hopes of bringing people closer together. Unfortunately, the lack of adherence to institutions and traditions has instead allowed people to drift apart rather than connect. It places the burden of finding meaning on the individual or family rather than on an established social group. In rejecting labels, we have lost some of the connectedness to others that marked previous generations. Now, in the middle years, many of us desire to recreate community.

THE CHANGING BLUEPRINT FOR WOMEN'S LIVES

In the changes, advancements, regressions, and rejections of the last forty-five years, we realize that the guidelines for women's roles are still fluid and uncertain. The old sex roles are gone, but no clear replacements have emerged.

Lydia was eager to discuss all the changes that she has been making and remembered the moment she first realized that there were rooms closed to her. "There weren't a lot of options and it really kind of limited our world to a man and children." Lydia recalled the book *Women's Room*.[9] "I remember reading that in my twenties, and it literally changed me. Anger came out and I was just enraged. I didn't realize how personalized it was for me. We grew up one way, and then we had all this other stuff going on, and it's been very complicated, and it's been great because there's been so many options, but it's been scary for us. . . . I don't want that fearfulness to rule my life, and I know I have to fight because that's what I grew up with."

Twenty years ago in psychology, a referral for therapy made to a woman psychologist was prefaced with the statement, "She's a woman *but* she is very good"—semiapologetic, requiring explanation. Even women seeking therapy went first to men, reflecting the same mistrust and low opinion of women that society had. Now, women like women better. This again mirrors an increase in our collective self-esteem. On the phone recently with a young woman I have never met, trying to help her find a good therapist, I gave her the name of a male colleague because he had the time, the gentleness, and the expertise needed for the problem she described. The woman called me back to tell me that, after thinking about it, she would prefer the name of a woman. Another example of change is that most women of my generation would agree that when our mothers (it would have been our mothers who kept appointments) took us to see a doctor when we were children and a woman walked out, we knew that she was the nurse. Our children do not immediately make those assumptions. My daughter Jenny worked in a lawyer's office during the summer of 1994 and was annoyed that the secretaries washed their own dishes and the boss did not. I thought it was more about power than gender, but she saw the inequality. I worked in a lawyer's office during the summer of 1960 and it never occurred to me to note the inequalities of gender or power; they were normal. In these ways, we have done well for our daughters.

We seem to have progressed from feeling comfortably second-rate to men to feeling uncomfortably second-rate, to attempts to be identical, and now we are at a confusing but creative time of trying to understand and value differences. One of the continuing distinctions is in life paths.

Mary Catherine Bateson wrote about life paths in the introduction to her book describing five women who "composed their lives":

Today, the material and skills from which a life is composed are no longer clear. It is no longer possible to follow the paths of previous generations. This is true for both men and women, but it is especially true for women, whose whole lives no longer need be dominated by the rhythms of procreation and the dependencies that these created, but who must still live with the discontinuities of female biology and still balance conflicting demands. Our lives not only take new directions; they are subject to repeated redirection, partly because of the extension of our years of health and productivity.[10]

Socially and economically, middle-class women are in positions to guide their own lives better than ever before, but today's lives often have an over-abundance of riches—many demands and commitments that are all important. Young people are taught that there is one model for a successful life and it includes early decision and commitment to one path. Women's lives are not necessarily focussed on one ambition; multiplicity of interests does not reflect inadequacy or lack of commitment. Instead, Bateson calls women's diversity "lives in which commitments are continually refocused and redefined."[11] Particularly relevant are Bernice Neugarten and Nancy Datan's examinations of personality development as it is intertwined with time. Time is an essential concept in the middle years. Time tells us when to get up, when to eat, when to go to the dentist for a cleaning, when to be grandparents, when to reach the pinnacle of success, when to be worried that we are old. Time also marks "time lived" and "time left," defining issues of adulthood that drive or inhibit creative growth. Neugarten and Datan use three sociological concepts: life time, social time, and historical time.[12]

Life time is age and, as such, relies on biological underpinnings. *Social time* is a dimension underlying age and influenced by cultural values, for example, the range of years when a girl is "marriageable." *Historical time* refers to the social, economic, and political events that influence life and gradually change social institutions.

Life Time

Life time refers to chronological age and is used to measure where we ought to stand on any number of physical, psychological, or cultural markers. Are we in our proper developmental niche? Life time is more helpful in describing child development where change is rapid, closely tied to chronological age, and directly intertwined with psychological change and cultural expectations. For adults, life time is useful in determining the average age for the onset of menopause or the age at which we collect Social Security. However, age is less useful for predicting adult psychological and social milestones. Most of the work that ties age to appropriate milestones has been based on men's patterns of living—in what order they do things and what they have accomplished—and does not have accurate application to the lives of women. Using a male measure, women wind up looking wrong. Women's psychological and social milestones are more often tied to social role choices than to age. At forty, some women may be at the top of their careers, but others may just be starting, changing, or slowing down to care for children. Still others may shift to part-time work to meet responsibilities of the middle years, such as caring for aging parents.[13] Even women with lifelong careers are rarely in an economic position to reassess work commitments by age forty, which is what the literature says that men do. Forty may feel like midlife at work to a man, but not necessarily to a woman. Women balance multiple roles and follow idiosyncratic paths. Unique patterns emerge, depending on the personal configuration of age at marriage, age at childbearing, having or not having children, stage of family life cycle, age entering the workforce, career, and method of balancing multiple responsibilities. Biology alone is insufficient to explain our lives. Chronological age focusses too heavily on biology, such as menopause and ending the reproductive years.[14] Chronological age alone does not reflect the patterns of women's lives.

Developmental markers vary in different cultures. For example, in this country it is not remarkably unusual for a forty-year-old woman to be pregnant with her first child, but it would be highly unlikely in others. Women now can have lives that include, as well as go beyond, sexuality and reproduction. Even reproductive desires seem to have changed. Nearly twice as many women born between 1945 and 1960 will never have children (16–17 percent) as compared to women born in the 1930s (8–9 percent). Also, women who do have children have one child fewer on the average than mothers born in the 1930s (2 to 3.2).[15] It may well be that the primary value of women was for so long dependent on their reproductive abilities and sexual attractiveness that chronological age was enough of a yardstick to measure value. The women I spoke with found other definitions of value, and these women—with children or without, married or not, gorgeous or plain—are hitting their stride.

Social Time

Social time refers to a dimension underlying age, for example, when a girl is marriageable. Social time divides ages into periods of time when society expects things to occur: we expect that women will raise children between certain ages, and if she has them much earlier or later, she is off-time; we consider a woman "young" during a certain phase of life, and "middle-aged" during another. This gives form to our cultural values as well. We are generally uncomfortable when we see ourselves off-time, either early or late, for major life events, such as becoming a grandmother, marrying, or making career moves. We have accepted cultural expectations, so socially determined perception of where we should be is important.[16] For example, Grace, at forty-five, has returned to college. She loves school but feels terribly old and "different." She also wonders what she will experience as the "new kid" at work when she graduates. Unfortunately, decisions on where we are "supposed to be" may cause us to feel personally off-time and embarrassed.

Historical Time

Historical time refers to the social, economic, or political events that influence our life course and gradually change social institutions. For example, in the early days of the women's movement (mid-1800s), Elizabeth Cady Stanton and others focussed on the sexual and social liberation of the individual woman, in addition to the right to vote, as the key to equality. They believed that gaining the right to vote would be only one step because after women gained the vote, the early feminist movement would lose steam. Indeed, the vote alone did not liberate women. People still believed that a woman's natural role was that of wife and mother, to be exercised only in the private sphere of the home as the guardian of the family's spiritual values. Therefore, in gaining the vote, it was popularly reasoned, women should bring their superior home-nurtured morality into the public arena and see to it that social reforms would protect the family. This emphasis on doing good for others led to a submergence of women's individual goals. On the positive side, when women did gain the vote, they worked toward the passage of infant care, health care, care of pregnant mothers, consumer protection, and other legislation. On the negative side, women neglected to use their vast political experience to gain office or build a political power base. This meant that no significant female voting bloc existed; politicians did not need to appeal to women. Elizabeth Cady Stanton's focus proved correct. The real obstacle to equality was not the vote but the division of lifestyles between men and women. Only when women became self-supporting, equal partners with men, as Stanton put it, would they be able to begin to exercise the hard-won right to vote in large numbers. It was changes in society that would change politics, not the other way around. Beginning in the mid-1960s, women moved to political activism, and this accounted for the growing power of women at the polls, and therefore an increase in status.[17]

The feminist movement has been stressful because it points out, for all to see, that women have not been welcome in many arenas of society. For those of us who had not figured it out on our own, feminism pointed out all the ways that women remained outside power. In any culture, the "right way" is defined by the majority, and whether the majority is constituted by greater numbers or more power, as in South Africa, majority thinking becomes the accepted way. We see it, we feel it, and we begin to believe that our ways are not just different but wrong or inferior.

CREATING NEW PATHS

All our commitments—the balancing of self and other, work and family, or an overcrowded schedule—stressful as they are, have enriched our lives. We are sophisticated jugglers. Roles shift again in the middle years; responsibilities need to be reviewed and rebalanced. By now we have the experience to think for ourselves. If we ask ourselves honestly, we see that we knew which commitments were right for us at each stage. At this time, we can create a path for the present, finally rejecting stereotypes or conventions if they don't work in our lives. Personality, family, and national and world events all become part of our psychological makeup. By implication, this also means that as the grown-ups, we can shape events which will mold the children to come.

Midlife is the time to listen to the accumulated experience of women before us—their victories and defeats. Whatever used to be the "right" way to do things, our own voices can guide mindful decisions based on the realities of our own lives. Yes, there have been contradictions throughout. These will continue. As May Sarton's writer, Hilary Stevens, says, "The women who have tried to be men have always lacked something: we have to rest on Sappho, Jane Austen, Colette . . . , we have to be *our selves*."[18]

NOTES

The quote in the chapter title is from a lecture given by Helen Keller in 1929.

1. Carl Jung, (1971), Marriage as a psychological relationship, in J. Campbell (Ed.), *The portable Jung* (New York: Viking), p. 165. Original work published 1931.

2. William Chafe, (1991), *The paradox of change: American women in the twentieth century* (New York: Oxford University Press), p. 152.

3. Ibid., p. 168.

4. Terri Orbuch and Lindsay Custer, (1995), The social context of married women's work and the impact on black and white husbands, *Journal of Marriage and the Family* 57:333–45.

5. Chafe, *Paradox of change*, p. 169.

6. Betty Friedan, (1983), *The feminine mystique* (New York: Dell).

7. Myra MacPherson, (1985), *Long time passing: Vietnam and the haunted generation* (New York: Doubleday), p. 35.

8. Paul Light, (1988), *Baby boomers* (New York: Norton), p. 19.

9. Her reference is to Marilyn French's 1977 novel, *The women's room*.

10. Mary Catherine Bateson, (1989), *Composing a life* (New York: Plume Press), p. 2.

11. Ibid., p. 9.

12. Bernice Neugarten and Nancy Datan, (1973), Sociological perspectives on the life cycle, in P. B. Baltes and K. W. Schaie (Eds.), *Life span developmental psychology: Personality and socialization* (New York: Academic Press).

13. Barbara Reinke, (1985), Psychosocial changes as a function of chronological age, *Human Development* 28:266–69.

14. Rosalind Barnett and Grace Baruch, (1978), Women in the middle years: A critique of research and theory, *Psychology of Women Quarterly* 3(2):187–98.

15. U.S. Census Bureau, Martin O'Connell, chief of the bureau's fertility statistics branch.

16. Neugarten and Datan, Life cycle.

17. Bella Abzug with Mim Kelber, (1984), *Gender gap* (Boston: Houghton Mifflin).

18. May Sarton, (1965), *Mrs. Stevens hears the mermaids singing* (New York: Norton), p. 112.

❖ 8 ❖

"ONCE YOU ARE REAL YOU CAN'T BE UGLY"
Authenticity

I will incline my ear to a parable; I will lay open my mystery to the music of a lyre.
  —Psalms 49:5

The payment for illusion? Despair.
  —Talmud: Pirke Avot

Authenticity and subordination are totally incompatible.
  —Jean Baker Miller, *Toward a New Psychology of Women*

The dilemma of authenticity is poignantly described in the children's book *The Velveteen Rabbit*. The rabbit is a little boy's Christmas present. He is all a rabbit should be—"fat and bunchy, with real thread whiskers, a new spotted coat, and ears lined with pink satin." The Skin Horse, who is the oldest and wisest toy in the nursery, becomes the rabbit's nursery mentor. One day, the rabbit asks him, "What is Real?"

"Real isn't how you are made," said the Skin Horse. "It's a thing that happens to you. When a child loves you for a long, long time, . . . then you become Real. . . . It takes a long time. That's why it doesn't often happen to people who break easily, or have sharp edges, or who have to be carefully kept. Generally, by the time you are Real, most of your hair has been loved off, and your eyes drop out and you get loose in the joints and very shabby. But these things don't matter at all, because once you are Real you can't be ugly, except to people who don't understand. . . . Once you are Real you can't become unreal again. It lasts for always."

The Rabbit sighed. He thought it would be a long time before this magic called Real happened to him. He longed to become Real, to know what it felt like: yet the idea of growing shabby and losing his eyes and whiskers was rather sad. He wished he could become it without these uncomfortable things happening to him.[1]

Ah, a midlife rabbit! Our eyes do not have to drop out, but we do have to allow ourselves the discomfort of not being too "carefully kept," which means letting go of the restrictions of being who we should be rather than who we are. We have been taught to be polite, to defer to others, and to fulfill their dreams rather than our own. We have been taught to be subordinate, economically inferior, and fearful, keeping us unreal and inauthentic. I have treated women who have learned to fake everything, from sexual pleasure to ideas and opinions. Authenticity, or becoming "Real," is the goal of all the efforts we put into reconnecting with ourselves, but it is not possible when we are too carefully kept.

THE RISK OF BEING VULNERABLE

To "become Real," or authentic, requires vulnerability. This is a necessary aspect of creative living. Every risk that we take to bring us closer to ourselves makes us vulnerable, because a risk, by definition, is a gamble. You can never truly be sure how a gamble will turn out. We are vulnerable because we go further into the unknown. The results may surprise, embarrass, or reward us. Whatever the outcome, we do not know it when we start out. The sense of being vulnerable is that of being undressed or exposed. Although we want to be known and understood, we also want to control how much of us is seen, by whom, and with what results.

Vulnerability is here in this writing. How much of me can be seen? As a therapist, clearly I remain in the shadows. That is an aspect of attending to others. Writing does not afford the same protection. An artist client described her struggle with feelings of exposure and vulnerability on the eve of an important show. She said that over the years she had learned to cope by being fully present at the creation of her art but becoming distant at the showing of her work. She protects herself by moving into dim light when people come to see the show.

The women I describe had to face being vulnerable. The thrill of breaking new ground, learning more about themselves, and doing more with their lives outweighed the risks, but could not eliminate the gamble. They took chances because of the inherent rewards in creative thought, spontaneity, discovery, and the possibility of leading the lives they had come to believe in. No matter how nicely decorated, a cage is still a cage.

These are ordinary women. They possess self-esteem and dozens of other good qualities, but have not been granted extraordinary gifts. They are also not dysfunctional, destroyed women. What makes them inspiring is that they continue to engage life, push further, and take some chances in order to make life a bit more of an adventure. There were essential elements in their searches to be authentic. All struggled to develop greater acceptance of self and others, more confidence in their judgment, and a healthy sense of entitlement. During the middle years, women are finally able to loosen overreactions and the desire to please others in favor of acceptance of self and others, let go of childhood insecurities in favor of confidence, and modify the instinct to always put the care of others before healthy entitlement.

ACCEPTANCE

A number of women said that they always had positive self-esteem but that they have come into something different at midlife: acceptance of themselves based on self-knowledge. Self-examination is frightening because we imagine we will learn all that is awful and nothing that is wonderful. Clinical experience has taught me that self-examination rarely turns out that way. Instead, in looking at ourselves and our lives we gain knowledge of overlooked strengths as well as deficits. Through increased self-discovery, women move to a compassionate acceptance of themselves based on openness to all aspects of themselves. They like the women they have become.

Self-examination→ Self-knowledge→ Self-acceptance

Women said things like, "This is me, even if I change some more. This is the most me I can be right now." "This is the package. I'm not going to mold myself to satisfy anyone else." Acceptance is not the same thing as complacency—we may want to continue to change forever—but it is a focus on who we are now and how we feel now, without the immediate urge to be different, feel different, do things differently. Acceptance is being okay with now. We recognize that there are limits to who we are and what we do, and to life itself. We acknowledge the finiteness of life and the inevitable limitations of our choices within that life as being human.

Acceptance is knowing and believing, really believing, that it is okay to be ourselves. Then we are free to allow others to be themselves. One woman said, "Acceptance. Accepting the present; I have always been very future oriented. Trying to live in the present, accepting that things don't happen because I will it so; accepting different opinions of people who are not like me; more accepting of my husband, of myself—you have to forgive yourself first."

Another voiced a similar idea in her own way: "I don't know which comes first. It's accepting that you have no frigging control over the kids anymore. They will do just what they will do, and that it's okay." A potter from Santa Cruz said, "It must be that our self-acceptance drives our acceptance of our children, because if you start to accept who you are, you lighten up a little bit. I was disappointed that [my daughter] was a complete nebbish in high school. I had such a great time in high school, and finally I woke up and said, who gives a horse's crap about high school? High school is nothing. Four lousy years and everyone makes so much about it." When we accept ourselves, we begin to accept others, not just give lip service to acceptance. We can see our children, our husbands, lovers, and family members, and accept them for the people they are. It is not going to kill us that they aren't the people that we had, at one time, wished them to be, imagined them to be, and hated them for not being.

Acceptance enables us to make changes or not. We become better able to face events as they exist and not distort situations with our wishes. Ideals and ambitions that were formed long ago in childhood do not necessarily have to be tossed aside, but can be updated in the face of new, overriding realities. A teacher in Evanston, Illinois, talked about giving up the "*House and Garden* life" after her divorce. It was a life that was her mother's dream for her.

Being the perfect wife and the perfect mother in the perfect world. . . . A challenge is over, but the other part is, my son does not like this house. This is a little cottage compared to where we lived before. He has a sense of this being a very diminished life. Well, in any case, he thinks this is just really impoverished and limited . . . but I find that I'm very happy with this—a scale of living that seems really humane and possible to me. . . . "Stuff" used to mean a lot more to me than it does now. It's a liberation, a relief. But it means that what I think [is] an enhancement in my life is a downturn for [my son's] life.

For me, it was years before I could accept the petty realities of life. I fought against taking time to clean, do laundry, or even be sick. These felt like interruptions to be minimized. It was only when I realized that chores are also part of my life, not interferences, that I was able to respect and do them.

Acceptance rooted in our lives now can continue to underscore our attitudes for the rest. It involves developing compassion for our younger selves. Rose, a psychologist now in her fifties, struggled during her twenties as a young, inept mother with four children under the age of five. But now she says, "I'm coming to terms with feelings of guilt, whatever I didn't do. It is right now for me. Like an acceptance, it was okay, I was a human being. I look at my kids. My kids like me. What is going on is a review of that."

Con, too, has begun to accept herself. She is, at forty-three, strikingly lovely and talented, and was written up in the art magazines for her recent work. Yet she lived for years with a sense that when she looked into a mirror, she could see scars on her face. Only in the last two years have the scars disappeared, as she began to grapple with memories of surviving incest. As Con gained a new, more complete understanding of herself, the old, injured images faded, and she accepted the lovely woman reflected in the mirror.

Patricia, a former businesswoman, also has enjoyed a new reaction to herself.

I will tell you unabashedly, for the first time, I was watching a video my daughter took of me at my retirement party. I saw a woman who isn't as thin as I would like her to be, but looking at her, listening to her, I came out and said to Stan, "If she were a friend of mine, or someone I met at a party, I'd like her. She's honest, she's not a hypocrite, she tries to have a good time." [When I was younger] I would never have been able to detach myself like that and look at myself, except to say, "Look at my nose, look at my hair, look at my dress." I admit that those thoughts went through as a first whiff, but [then] I thought, "She's okay."

Acceptance for Claire, now forty-seven, involved some basic self-discovery about sexuality. When she reflected back on her life, she saw herself as always angry, but she never quite knew why.

What else do I want, I would think to myself. I didn't know what else I wanted, and it wasn't until I came out [as a lesbian] seven years ago that I realized what it is that I want. You know, there's just this opening and freeing feeling. . . . I spent some time regretting: "I wish I would have known this earlier about myself." But I really believe totally that you have to go through certain experiences, whatever life gives you, to become the person that you are.

I can do anything that I want to do; even if I'm scared and terrified, I can do it. I just gotta sit down and methodically go through how I think. . . . Even if I don't have the answers, I'm still gonna go for it. If I feel that inherent strength deep inside of me, that it feels right, then I'm just gonna do it. I'm just gonna keep working in that direction because I believe in God. I believe that if I am totally open to what's out there for me, it's gonna start happening. Just opening up that door and not being closed to faith has just done incredible things. And it happens every day of my life.

Acceptance for Ginny, a community organizer and a woman still struggling to keep her failing marriage together, came with the understanding that she thought well of herself. "I like me. If he doesn't, then he probably should leave. I won't let him treat me badly because I'm not the woman in his imagination."

Endorsement is an early and continuing part of the venturing journey. Usually we fight hard to change ourselves and others, to be different, better, thinner, prettier, and smarter. Ambitions are great. Change is essential. Dreams are necessary. But with it all, we find a greater peace if we hold on to a basic satisfaction with ourselves and life.

A level of honesty never before possible has become available to many women. Nan said, "All the small lies I ever told myself don't work so well anymore." Grace said, "I can't lie anymore. And I'm not young anymore and I'm realizing, this is who I am, way older than all the models and most of the movie stars. You don't even listen to the same music. All that gave me courage to stop pretending." We face ourselves and our lives, and we accept the limitations. That makes honesty easier: there is less to hide, we have already examined our skeletons and found them manageable, we can figure out who we are and be ourselves. This includes all the good in ourselves. We can allow others to know us or not. We move another inch closer to freedom.

CONFIDENCE IN OUR JUDGMENT

Confidence matures, based on experience and self-knowledge. What we call confidence is closely related to trust, but trust has essential roots in early experiences with a quality of belief and mutuality. Confidence is all that plus adult experience—a mature self-trust, belief in ourselves in addition to well-placed faith in other people. Confidence is based on determination, certainty, and conviction. It is another gift we receive as a result of our reconnection to ourselves. Confidence rests on the belief that we are able to take risks based on our solid judgment. We believe that when we fall down, we will be able to get up and go on. Lynn said, "If that next step doesn't work out, then there'll be another one that does. I think I was not at all sure of myself. I think I've always acted in the world like I was sure of myself. I know I have. I made a point of it, and I've convinced other people, but now I'm really pretty sure that I can do what comes. And that's a new knowledge and sense of hope. I can do it. . . . It's confidence."

Confidence reassures us that we can be vulnerable and survive if we are wounded by taking risks. Carolyn, who has been hearing impaired since birth, explains, "There will be a lot of situations where I can't hear. That's just the way it's going to be. It's not so frightening." Carolyn worked hard to reach the point of feeling good enough about herself to make mistakes without being devastated and to refrain from overly protecting herself, for example, by avoiding people or noisy social situations. Carolyn said that her confidence came from liking herself, feeling competent, and knowing that she could come back to situations that had failed and make them work better.

Confidence, then, is the belief that we can continue despite setbacks. We can go on, after making the human, normal, foolish mistakes that we must make in order to grow. We have the ability to correct, to persist, and to work toward a better way, without expecting perfection. Perfection isn't human. Confidence also includes an inner certainty that as we experience the discomfort of change, we can hold onto an internal continuity that reassures and stabilizes us.

Confidence is also that simple, wonderful belief that life's tasks can be mastered as they arise. Elaine, now divorced after many years of marriage, expressed it well:

I can fill the air in my tires. There's no piece of the daily business of running the household that I can't do or figure out how to get . . . done. I used to really hate talking on the phone. I still do, and I give the impression of being very curt because I want to get off so fast. And now, I have to make all the phone calls myself and all the elaborate arrangements for babysitters. . . . That's really trivial. I hate it, and I can do it now, and at the end, I think, well, I did that okay.

She has come to trust her ability to take care of kids, chores, cars, and illnesses, even though she has not found perfection or the magic that will make the kids stop fighting or keep the car from breaking down. Nor has she discovered the secret to an orderly life. Rather, she trusts herself to take care of the disorder in an acceptable, mature, grown-up manner.

There is no speaking up and no taking action without self-confidence. Studies that have followed the same women, first as college graduates, later as young adults, and again at approximately forty-three, found that traditional femininity, which had increased after college, decreased at midlife, and at that time confidence rose. About life in the early forties, the women said that they were "being my own person; feeling more confident; having a wider perspective; focusing on reality and meeting the needs of the day without being too emotional about them; having influence in my community or area of interest; feeling my life is moving well; feeling secure and committed; feeling a new level of productivity or effectiveness; feeling powerful; and having interest in things beyond my own family."[2]

Melanie said that her experience with the video camera demonstrated that "I trusted my judgment better, I trusted myself better, I valued myself more, I respected myself more, because I was dealing with losing everything." Melanie could not give in to anyone else's needs one more time to keep the peace. This decision was based on confidence in her judgment and not allowing anyone to override her experience or assessment of the problem. She explained her understanding of it to Tim, her long-time partner, and he explained his different understanding. She had to choose between his meaning and her meaning. After talking and arguing, she still believed and followed her view. Later, when others agreed with her, she did not feel victorious. She had not been battling for domination; rather, it had been a fight for the right to exercise her own judgment.

Claire illustrates the attitude needed to take risks based on personal judgment. She quit her job to open a shop and describes the daily ventures she takes in her business: "I really believe that when your mind and heart are just open . . . to [listening] to that voice inside. . . . When something doesn't feel right, we just don't do it. And if it feels right, then we do it. And if it feels right, and we don't have the money, then we do part of it and go back to it. . . . I really do trust myself. . . . That voice inside is really worth listening to. So I stop and wait." Claire's confidence in her judgment allows her to continue to take risks. Today, the store is thriving in Chicago.[3]

Confidence reminds us that we can and will make mistakes, but we will not be stopped by errors. Margaret, a former client, was absolutely terrified of making mistakes. To Margaret, a mistake meant it was all over, there was no way to fix it. In therapy, where we often examined the issue of making mistakes, we developed a standing joke: "If you fell down outside in the snow, would you yell for your husband to bring a tent so you could stay there forever, or would you pick yourself up and climb out?" It was a rhetorical question, of course, yet so many women are like Margaret, fearful of making mistakes because they believe that they would be bound forever to the results. Margaret's associations led to memories of her mother, who would say, "You made your bed, now lie in it." I heard a complementary quip several months later in a discussion group I led: "If you lay down with dogs, you get up with fleas." We have so many restrictive warnings to stay "carefully kept," so as adults we have a lingering belief that we are morally obligated to live with naive, youthful, or simply stupid mistakes.

When we fall down, we can get up. Gymnasts learn not to fear the floor. Skaters learn to fall to the ice. Confidence, then, is enough belief in our judgment to act, whether we succeed or fail, and to make corrections.

ENTITLEMENT

"I didn't feel entitled about anything before and suddenly I started to feel like I was. . . . I used to feel grateful for anything that went well and hunkered down when it didn't." At some point in each of the women's lives, just being alive stopped being enough. Melanie, who made the statement above, remembered, "I would say, at least I'm alive. Okay, for God's sake, there's more to life than just being alive! . . . To go through life grateful that you don't have cancer—that's me. Or to be grateful that your children didn't get hit by a car. That's how I've lived—with all these fingers in the dike. There's a lot that happens before you get cancer and die." Most of us were raised to be grateful for what we have, to be sure not to put our own needs before those of others, and to be unselfish and never greedy.

You may have cringed when you saw the heading of this section, "Entitlement." It draws attention to "me": "I want," "I deserve." It feels selfish and greedy. Children, not women, shriek, "What about me!" The value of women has always come from our talent to know others, feel for others, and facilitate others. Those are wonderful qualities. They keep us in touch with our emotional life and the feelings of others; they keep us close to the people we love. However, these qualities also keep us away from thinking too much about what we want. Entitlement raises the nasty question of self-interest. It puts each of us into the picture—right there with everybody else's needs and wants. Not *instead of* the others, but *in addition to* the others. Unfortunately, when we put ourselves into the equation, it can feel like we are pushing someone else out.

I am endlessly amazed at the difficulty women seem to have with the phrase "I want." For example, Laura, forty-five, attended school with a friend of mine, so I had met her years ago. She was intimidating, even with her giggle and soft voice. She had a reputation as hardworking and very competent, as quite a star. After graduate school, she and her husband moved back to the South, where she directed an innovative hospital program. Later, she moved to a prestigious university position. I saw her from time to time and knew that the people who worked for her at the university thought she was wonderful and the programs ran well, and I envied the ease with which she seemed to manage the internal politics. During these same years, she wrote professional articles and book chapters and became involved in a consulting business. Last year, she left to manage her own consulting firm and begin some new projects. When I interviewed her for this book, I was surprised to find that Laura's view of herself contrasted sharply with my view of her. Yet she said, in all honesty,

If I think about where I am right now . . . the [psychological work of the] last couple of years has been to be able to take the risks required to do what I wanted to do. I had to get stronger to make the choices to say, "I don't want this, I do want that." The last year has been about leaving the school and not working so hard, which is just a beginning. [I'm] trying to get rid of the "supposed to do" that kept me, partly as an excuse, from doing the things I wanted to do. Now I have done that. Whether I can proceed and do what I want to do is an issue.

What had stopped her?

I don't think I felt good enough about myself to take those risks. It feels very much like a risk for me to even say, "This is what I want to go after." That's not part of my upbringing, where I might say, "Gee, I really want that," and go after it. I've never done that in my life. . . . I come from a family background that was poor and where people didn't see themselves as having a lot of options, having no rights, socialized as a southern white female. Even now, spending money on myself, well . . . (laugh)

Even saying I can make this company work or saying I don't need to work eighty hours a week, giving myself the permission to say [that] these are my dreams and I'm going to try to make this happen, feels very risky to me. My whole life has been, well, things just happen, rather than saying, "This is what I want," and going after it.

There were a number of events in Laura's life that allowed her to begin to make changes. "The situation got so unbearable at the school that I had to get out. So it was unbearable *and* I had become clearer about other things I wanted to do. As the issues became clearer to me, in terms of cultural and women's issues, and my experience . . . was so different from the provost, it put us in opposition." She had encountered her own ideas and those of others with whom she worked closely. "I was supporting things that were increasingly important to me that he really didn't understand— that he saw as marketing. I became, not by choice, the leader of the op- position . . . ; it made me see things that I could have ignored on my own, and then I had to take a stand. . . . I got caught in their battle."

The situation seemed to crystallize for Laura at an administrative session.

Sitting at that meeting made me realize how hopeless the whole situation was and that nothing was going to change. I had been quite vocal about the things I believed in and the things I believed needed to happen, and sitting at that meeting, I was overwhelmed with the hopelessness of the whole situation . . . ; they had no respect for what we were trying to do, no real respect for that. . . . It felt so overwhelming to me, so hopeless, and they didn't get the point. I kept crying. I couldn't stop. . . . I just cried. It felt very personal. If I could have not gone back, I would have. I had a month off. If I could have figured out a way never to set foot in that building again, I would have done it.

Laura had changed by reconnecting to her beliefs about cultural diversity and women's issues at the university. "It was a conservative, rule-oriented position, more than I am. . . . I was getting cast into this role that I really didn't want. Initially it wasn't a big deal. I could do the position in a way that was comfortable to me. It went more conservative, rule oriented."

Now, with her own company, "I can run [it] in a way that is compatible and interesting to me. I started feeling good about myself again, finding some kind of validation. Looking back, I think I was much too critical of myself. I felt like I hadn't done a good enough job at standing up for women's issues. I felt like a failure at that. I was very much aware of that. Now, I don't think so, but at the time, I felt I did a terrible job."

Gabby said, "I had gotten to the point where I could say, 'Wait a minute, my turn is the front of the line right now. It's not your turn any longer.' Generally, that's what the children say. But I also have to sometimes do that with friends. I don't do it as much as I should, but it's a goal I'm working towards. . . . That may have to do with the sort of movement into finding what's right for me." She realized, too, that she wanted fun back in her life. In spite of financial uncertainty, Gabby went ahead with plans made a year and a half earlier to visit the Southwest. Her girlfriend assumed that they would have to call the vacation off. "I debated back and forth: Is it on? Is it off? I can't leave the children. This is too much stress. I just don't have the money. And I just said, 'Yes I can; I'm going.' It was a great trip. . . . It didn't make any sense . . . I wanted it, and that's good enough. So, I did it."

It was difficult for Gabby to think about her wants without experiencing fears about her family being hurt or deprived of time and money. In these dilemmas, we see how difficult it becomes for women to acknowledge what they want and then to express their needs without feeling selfish. Gabby may have been able to address the problem more directly than many women because she had been raised by women who were "tough cookies" and she had always worked and made money. Nan was very direct also: "I don't deserve to be treated badly. I will not be kept waiting for an hour in a doctor's office without saying something. My time is valuable, too. I won't be scolded—not by my husband, kids, or anyone else. I won't have people in my life who treat me with disrespect. I'm not a fool. I won't let myself in for that shit anymore."

Other women, like Mary Sue, at times resorted to manipulation, a tool of the weak, in order to get what they wanted. Mary Sue was raised in a home where social contacts meant everything and women had very sharply defined roles that were traditionally feminine. She said that she is "working on communicating what I need. I was miserable at it; now I'm only bad at it. The way I was reared, some of it was a given, the rest you manipulated. You manipulate [to get] what you want; you don't come right out and ask for it."

Entitlement takes courage because when we speak up, knowing that each of our voices will differ from other voices, we also recognize that others prefer us to remain caring and cooperative. To speak in our own voices is a risk, but to remain silent means to remain inauthentic. To collude in devaluing ourselves eliminates us as deserving care. At midlife, it is no longer worth the peace.

One reaction that stands in the way of acceptance, confidence, and entitlement is guilt. Guilt about putting ourselves first, guilt about wants, and guilt about being a greedy, selfish child. Melanie remembered many times that guilt haunted her: "When I got divorced, I was sure I would get hit by a train." We feel guilt when we want something that might be in our best interest but not necessarily in the best interest of someone else. Then we feel guilty when we get things we want or when we win, because we imagine someone else has lost. We may be able to circumvent guilt by intensely caring for others, but the danger is that our generosity has strings attached. In Disney movies, good people are rewarded and bad people are punished. In real life, often unknowingly, we expect to be rewarded for being good and helpful. And we get resentful and hurt when care is not returned. We are bitter that others have not taken good care of us. But what we have done is not true giving; it is a roundabout way of trying to get something without directly asking. The women interviewed have realized that true gifts do not have invisible strings attached. On the other hand, these women have also learned that they do not need to always give; sometimes they trade, and sometimes they simply receive. They have learned to take action to insure justice or fairness; no matter how good they have been, fairness is not guaranteed.

The ability to care for others will always be among the greatest gifts women possess. Generosity toward others is a strength, but not when it is extended instead of generosity toward self. We do not have the right to expect everything to be done for us or to expect others to subjugate themselves for our needs, but healthy entitlement means that we certainly have the right to equal give-and-take.

One antidote to guilt is development of healthy narcissism, or self-love. In previous chapters, we examined the ways that women grow in relation to others and the difficulty of balancing attention to others with attention to ourselves. In our middle years, it becomes more possible to use our gifts of understanding and connection for our own creative living. Gifts that have been used for years in an outward direction, we can now turn inward. When we were younger and hypersensitive to others, we may have surrendered ourselves. Loving others, we failed to adequately love ourselves.

With only a connection to and love for others, and little for ourselves, creativity is not possible. Midlife is an opportune time to attend to ourselves because outside connections are already in transformation—kids are leaving, we are aging, parents are ailing—and we are aware as never before of limited time. But one of the questions women ask is how to maintain the balance of attending to self and attending to others. Studies don't give us the "right" answer. They only tell us what other people are doing. The question of balancing attention between others and ourselves remains central during most of our lives. The specific answer depends on our age, life circumstance, family constellation, and personality needs—all of which change with time. We ask the same questions; it's the answers that change.

Attention to one's self, entitlement, or normal narcissism, is love of self. Self-love is balanced by love of others. That blend leads to intimacy and love as evidenced by closeness, affection, cooperation, and dependability. Of course, there are abnormal extremes. Narcissism, at one end, becomes an excessive absorption with one's self. At the other extreme, loving others creates an inattention to one's self in favor of others, with accompanying feelings of victimization and estrangement from oneself. A study of forty-three-year-old women who fell at either end of the self-related or other-related continuum showed that those women who scored high on the self-directed, or narcissistic, side of the prototype had qualities of hypersensitivity, lowered empathy, and willfulness. This lowered the control of their own aggression and sexuality and led to self-indulgence. But the women who had healthy levels of narcissism had qualities of autonomy, norm questioning, independence, and work orientation, which allowed creativity, satisfaction, and achievement.[4] These women experienced a harder time in their twenties because they were less conforming and more introspective than the others. They struggled to balance career and family. But in their forties, these autonomous and nontraditional women flourished because the inner world of ideas remained available to them.[5] The other-directed women showed little abnormality. They were straightforward and giving, socially competent, dependable, controlled, ready to accept life's demands, and attentive to interpersonal relationships, but not creative.[6] This study reminds us that creativity requires attention to self. An emphasis on others can create a stable life, but not a new one.

Increasingly as we age, we see ourselves as less sensitive to and less controlled by other people's demands and expectations. We are less interested in relationships that are obligatory rather than reciprocal. The direction of change is toward attending more to ourselves and desiring increased time for ourselves.[7] An increase in healthy narcissism gives us independence and freedom from the opinions of others, allowing creativity. For many of the women presented here, narcissism means feeling entitled to good things in life rather than merely making the best of every situation; feeling that it's okay to get their own way once in a while rather than accommodating others; acting instead of reacting; having views and needs, even when it inconveniences others; and learning to say, "I want," rather than always being grateful for not having cancer or not being run over by a car. We learn what we want when we recall our own voices, half-buried under other people's wants and needs, and bring those values and ideas to light.

NOTES

Quote in chapter title is from Margery Williams, *The velveteen rabbit or how toys become real* (see n. 1).

1. Margery Williams, (1985), *The velveteen rabbit or how toys become real* (New York: Doubleday), pp. 16–17.

2. Ravenna Helson and Geraldine Moane, (1987), Personality change in women from college to midlife, *Journal of Personality and Social Psychology* 53(1):181.

3. Claire asked that her story be dedicated to the memory of Aunt Kitty.

4. Paul Wink, (1991), Self- and object-directedness in adult women, *Journal of Personality* 59:769–91.

5. Paul Wink, (1992), Three types of narcissism in women from college to mid-life, *Journal of Personality* 60 (1):24–26.

6. Wink, Self- and object-directedness.

7. Bertram Cohler and Robert Galatzer-Levy, (1990), Self, meaning, and morale across the second half of life, in R. Nemiroff and C. Colarusso (Eds.), *New dimensions in adult development* (New York: Basic Books), pp. 214–59.

❖ 9 ❖

"Finding a Fortune in the Lining of an Old Coat"
Aggression and Creativity

People call me a feminist whenever I express sentiments that differentiate me from a doormat or a prostitute.
  —Rebecca West

Fair—this word is to be used only in reference to a carnival-type event and not as an expression of justice; for not only is such usage unpleasant but also, I assure you, quite useless.
  —Fran Lebowitz

Yesterday I dared to struggle.
Today I dare to win.
  —Bernadette Devlin

There are normal identity shifts during the middle years that enhance our opportunities to live creative lives. One important development is the emergence of healthy, ordinary aggression, which we can harness to work effectively for us. We make the most of our aggression when we are able to link the available energy to our creative attitudes. This combination fuels our actions.

Growth is easier when change happens naturally, when new aspects of ourselves gently unfold, and when we welcome the change. Growth is difficult when we fight against change and refuse to accept emerging aspects of ourselves. We are most apprehensive when we fear that change will take us too far away from our most basic sense of ourselves. Who have I become? It is frightening to think that we could become women who are foreign to the deepest knowledge we have of ourselves. Yet, in order to remain psychologically alive, we must allow new behaviors, like assertiveness and aggressiveness, to emerge. Identities that may have been complete when we were in our twenties need revision in our forties and fifties.

Aggression and anger are not the same thing. Anger is a feeling, an emotion, whereas assertiveness and aggressiveness refer to action. But many women believe that merely feeling angry leads to action. "Carriers of fire" is an expression that refers to the ability of whoever carries a flame to use it for creation or destruction. Anger is fire; we can carry it to fuel our creative lives, or we can reduce our lives to ashes. When we feel angry, we experience both the freedom and the danger.

The changes that occur in the midlife years are not really the creation of new personalities, but rather a step in the journey where we uncover attributes that have been buried in the lives we have led. Finding our misplaced selves, nourishing the unused bits and pieces of identity, becomes another way we continue to develop a creative approach to the years that lie ahead.

TRAPPED BY ANGER

All the psychology textbooks simply list anger as one of the basic emotions, yet it never seems quite that ordinary when we feel angry. When we are angry, we experience ourselves as dangerous, destructive, abnormal, or unusual. Anger frightens us and others; that is why so many people avoid it. Over the years, we begin to think that anger is unacceptable in women—unless we are defending others, especially children. Then, because the anger serves someone else, it becomes acceptable. We are admired when we protect our children or ridiculed as overprotective, but the anger is understood. People are not as agreeable when anger serves our own interests.

Anger is less acceptable in women than in men. No one likes to believe that the hand that rocks the cradle is shaking from rage. Society wants to believe that we are always *only* nurturing and caring, as if care, love, and anger cannot exist in the same person. There are old stories that describe women's destructiveness. Delilah betrayed Sampson, cut off his hair, sapped his strength, and led him to destruction; sirens lure men to death on the sea; and myths describe vaginal teeth that castrate men. Angry women are pictured as destructive, aggressive, and castrating. Fear of women arises out of the fact that, in most societies, women care for and raise children. Mothers are very important in young lives and continue to loom in our psyches as all-powerful. We depended on our caretakers, usually mother, for survival. This power had to be dealt with emotionally, and one very effective way of lessening power is to disparage the holder.[1]

The status of women in this country, and in most others, has evolved into an economically and politically weaker position. We have always been in subordinate positions to men in areas of power in this society, and this affects our feelings about the expression of anger. Our reactions to anger reflect societal views. Jean Baker Miller writes that in response to living in an inferior position, women tend to have the inner beliefs that reflect lower status.[2] These beliefs make it difficult to feel angry.

The first belief is "I am weak." The weakness begins to feel inherent rather than a result of position. This sense of weakness stamps out anger because women fear revenge from the stronger elements in society. Lori came in to my office sobbing because her ex-husband had threatened to take away the children if she pursued legal action to collect back child support payments. The threat and the belief that he could somehow win were enough to make her seriously consider backing down. She felt weak—not because of anything she had done and not because he had a good legal case, but simply from a fear that he was stronger and more aggressive than she. It took time for her to get angry, but when she did, she felt stronger.

The second inner belief is "I am unworthy," which is also very effective in smothering anger, because when we feel unworthy, self-hatred deepens. Gloria was so grateful to get a job at fifty after her company closed that she did everything she was told, no matter how ridiculous. She was the sixteenth office worker in seven years, so she knew her boss would be demanding. Gloria even knew that a monthly lunch club of ex-secretaries existed, but she needed a job and was determined to please her boss. He yelled instead of talking. His demands escalated weekly. She was allowed no phone calls, even if she was on a lunch break, no radio, and no conversations with customers who came through the building. Next, rules were instituted about what articles were allowed on top of her desk. All work was redone several times to strange specifications. Gloria did not think she could get another job, and she could not seem to please her boss. She became very frightened, but she hated herself instead of being angry at him for the ways that he mistreated her. She was not sure she deserved good treatment. His behavior escalated. He lectured her on prayer and other personal topics as well as the usual diatribes about work. Gloria began to look for a new job after he threw the telephone directory at her.

Women are often afraid that expressing anger will disrupt relationships, at home or at work, and many women depend on husbands or employers for economic security, so there is a realistic fear when these relationships are upset by anger. Ironically, being in a continually subordinate position is enough to generate anger.

The third inner belief that evolves from being in a subordinate position is "I have no right to be angry." This may be the most pervasive and destructive belief of them all. If we have no right to feel angry, then feeling angry will intensify our sense of defectiveness, irrationality, and worthlessness. Diane has two teenagers—good kids, but noisy, sloppy, and careless with her things. When the oldest borrowed her favorite earrings and lost one, Diane cried. She felt that she had made a mistake in lending her jewelry, effectively obliterating the appropriate anger that her older daughter's carelessness deserved.

Sherry's story demonstrates how anger can trap and free a woman. Sherry, now forty-eight, had spent much of her life feeling angry.

I was in a marriage for twenty-one years. I got married at eighteen, and hindsight showed me that I got out of my parents' home because there was abuse there, from my father to me, and I'm not even sure of all of it at this point. I just remember pieces. I didn't realize it then, so I got married young and I married somebody who was very much like my parents, again not realizing it until the marriage was over. My parents are both very angry people. He was an alcoholic, she was always on pills.

Sherry had gone directly from her parent's angry, destructive house to being a wife, but she had no idea, at age eighteen, what constituted a marital partnership.

"And I was filling this role as wife and mother, and I was so distracted by what I was doing, to take care . . . I have three sons to take care of and they're wonderful . . . that I lost track of who needs you. I didn't know who I was. Friends would say to me, 'Well, what do you want to do when your kids are all grown and away at school?' I didn't have a clue until I was thirty-one."

She and her husband divorced after more than twenty years together.

He and I never really had this equal partnership, even when I began working. I didn't make anywhere near the salary he did, so I was not as important as he was. I had two full-time jobs; what I was doing outside the house and inside the house. Everything was always his way. And something inside of me was hating this for years. I walked around as a very angry individual. I think if you ever interviewed any of my friends that knew me in New York while I was married, they would classify me as a very unhappy, angry woman . . . and it was true. . . . I had a house in the suburbs. . . . What else do I want, I would think to myself. . . . I couldn't really express my angers and resentments 'cause they were put down all the time. So, it just kind of grew in me.

Sherry was seething and assumed that she was simply an "angry person," never recognizing that the anger had developed, in good measure, from her being embedded in destructive situations.

We have come to know anger as destructive and aggressive, yet it does not have to be such. Normal people have a range of emotions, including anger. Life presents us with situations that elicit many emotions, and when we fail to show authentic feelings and reactions, we create psychological problems. Our trust of our own experience keeps us grounded, certain, and complete. If we are not permitted to have our own experiences, then we are disconfirmed as people. If anyone takes away our experiences and the feelings engendered by them, we are truly diminished.

When there is an essential inequality, relationships cannot be based on openness and reciprocity; rather, they operate on deception and manipulation. Safety and equality allow open disagreement, but that requires that women assume that their own needs have validity and proceed to explore and state them openly. Of course, this may be experienced as creating conflict, but how else can we be known and our needs be understood and fulfilled? Unknown will remain unfulfilled.

Our generations of women received mixed messages about our own growth and development. We were taken seriously only to a point—when our goals were to be able to earn a living if our husbands got sick, to seek work that provided security, to work hours that complemented children's schooling, and to take as few risks as possible. The career discussions that I remember in my own home all seemed to end with "Learn to type."

Instead of the pain of growth and self-analysis, we were encouraged to learn how to form and support relationships. So we learned the pain associated with fear of loss. We came to fear that self-absorption and growth would doom relationships. To avoid isolation, abandonment, loss of love and connectedness, Jean Baker Miller insists that women do two things: one, we divert ourselves from an exploration and expression of needs because we do not want to be in conflict with people and institutions. Second, we transform our needs. We fail to perceive our needs as such. We begin to think that our needs are the same as those expressed by our husbands, partners, family, children, co-workers, and bosses. When we satisfy the needs of others, then we are satisfied and fulfilled—for a time.[3] Over time, their needs become ours, and we attempt to carry them out. Somehow it is not good enough if it is our need—it must be his need or her need or work or favors. This works for a long time.

But as we grow older, children can do more for themselves, we mature, and we see more clearly how completely we justify all that we do. Instead of, "I want new shoes," we turn it into, "I need new shoes for work." Instead of admitting to fatigue and relaxing after a long day's work, Sara says that she feels sick and Marilyn drinks, because they cannot stop work in any other way. In their minds, if they still are alert, they should put in a few more hours of work. Self-confidence helps us to be able to express ourselves authentically. Otherwise, we substitute justification for expression of our wants and needs, as if our own ideas, needs, and wants are bogus. When we justify our wants and needs, we do not feel guilty. We remain selfless and innocent. We lose sight of what we want by the distance we put between our wants and ourselves. Unless it is productive, or work, or for the kids or for the family, our needs do not count.

Just as the Eskimos have many words for snow because it is integral to their life, we have developed many ways to repackage anger into a more acceptable form. Sara concentrated on how it could have been worse. "Sure, I was beaten, but no bones were broken." Melanie used to focus on what she had rather than on what she lost, "At least I don't have cancer!" Phyllis redirected her anger from the legitimate object to someone else with whom it was less dangerous to be angry. She did not scream at her boss; she yelled at her husband. Sherry unknowingly developed an elaborate method. Terrified of anger, she avoided her own emotion, and in the process, encouraged anger in others, then reacted to them and felt victimized. Olivia distorted situations in order to feel justified in her anger.

No one can give us freedom; we have to take it. Sometimes, getting good and angry helps to get us moving. Anger can wrench us away from others in a healthy way so that we can have the distance required to begin to inquire into ourselves instead of into others.

FREED BY ANGER

In *The Dance of Anger*, Harriet Goldhor Lerner writes that,

anger is a signal, and one worth listening to. Our anger may be a message that we are being hurt, that our rights are being violated, that our needs or wants are not being adequately met, or simply that something is not right. Our anger may tell us that we are not addressing an important emotional issue in our lives, or that too much of our self—our beliefs, values, desires, or ambitions—is being compromised in a relationship. Our anger may be a signal that we are doing more and giving more than we can comfortably do or give. Or our anger may warn us that others are doing too much for us, at the expense of our own competence and growth.[4]

One reason that anger appears during the middle years is that we are involved in the work of mourning. Anger often marks change and means that a separation has begun—a separation from a person, an idea, or an old view of life. It is a normal emotional response, simultaneously an emotional acknowledgment of change and a protest against it. Gabby mentioned that after she decided to divorce, she was surprised because she "became very angry and I kept wondering where does this rage come from. . . . Once I had made the decision to start, then I was just racked by rage and then racked by grief." The anger was important in mourning her dead marriage. The anger comes with the letting go, as we begin to feel the change deeply.

Sherry described the usefulness of anger in getting her life on track. In her late thirties, she had taken a secretarial job at a fine university because her son wanted to go to school there and they would save a great deal of money if she was an employee, but four years later, after her marriage had ended, she was hating every minute of it—yet her son wanted to continue in graduate school.

There was a fundamental change deep inside me that, I don't know, I think it was a lot of anger in there. I just could not continue being manipulated and pushed around. I had just gotten out of a long marriage where there was a lot of manipulation and pushing around, and I had reached my limit. I couldn't do it anymore. . . . The anger helps separate . . . ; it propelled me right out of there, and once that negative door closed, shortly thereafter, the positive one started opening. . . . Something happened inside of me. It was a feeling . . . that I knew I could not continue here.

Sherry thought about her future. "Am I going to retire from this place, this prison that I'm working in? Something just fundamentally shifted in here."

Later, Sherry realized that some of her hatred for the job was old anger from her marriage. Now that she feels free, she is trying to let go of old hurts and resentments. "I'm trying to get myself into a place where I can learn how to forgive, and that's a big one."

The anger that allowed Sherry to leave her job was only partly created by the school's atmosphere. She had been angry long before she went to work at the university. Sherry's experience with anger is not uncommon. Often it is not possible to fully feel anger until we are in a place that is safer than the original environment. Sherry had lived in angry environments for most of her life. Only after her divorce did she feel better. When school politics made her angry, she attacked the new event with the force called up from all the old situations. The anger was useful because it allowed her to move in directions closer to meeting her own needs.

Carol, who works with the elderly, was even more articulate about anger. She saw anger as useful when it did not become overwhelming and threaten her view of herself.

I get angry. I was very angry many times at the company. I got very angry; that's why I left there. They were screwing me over. When I get into situations where I'm angry all the time, I begin to think that's who I am, and then I need to get out of it . . . because I'm angry too much. I don't want to see myself that way, and I don't think it's fundamentally accurate. Anger is very mobilizing. I learned that from working with old people. I'd much rather be an angry old person than a depressed old person. You survive much longer, you get what you want . . . so it probably mobilized me in the same way.

Learning from feeling angry at situations or people that hurt us is only half the freedom. We can learn from being appropriately angry at ourselves, too. Nine summers ago, a friend suggested that I leave my raft, the only prize I had ever won in a raffle, in a shed on my property for the week because we were coming back on the following Friday. I remember thinking that it was a bad idea because the lock was missing, but it was easy. I wanted to believe that my raft would be safe. Of course, my raft was stolen. I was furious at myself. I knew better and did not pay attention to my own knowledge. The experience was very powerful for me because it drove home, *finally*, that I did not want to sink in anybody else's ship. I wanted to be the captain of my own ship if I had to take the risk of sinking in it. I had already figured out that I was going to make mistakes, but it was the raft that made me realize how important it is to listen to myself and make my own mistakes, not someone else's. If I hadn't been as angry, I would never have known that.

It was useful for me to get angry because I decided to trust myself more. If I had used the anger only to beat myself up, it would have been useless. This way, the anger allowed me to function more autonomously, not follow anyone else, and not blame others. It is not the experience of anger per se but what it allows us to do that is important. We can become more determined than ever to follow our own instincts.

The women I spoke with all made mistakes, plenty of them. Just like everybody else, they got angry at themselves and at others. What makes them special, and can make anyone special, is that they used what they learned. When they made a mistake, they learned from it. Blame is a waste of time and energy. Anger has its uses. It sends us messages. Women become more creative when they stop turning away from the messages and instead listen to them, honestly examine the situations and themselves, and attempt to act differently the next time.

WE CAN LEARN NEW TRICKS

For years, adulthood was ignored as a time of growth—not only by researchers, but also by those of us approaching maturity. How many of us looked ahead, except to vaguely imagine a husband, children, or job? When we were teenagers and continuing into our twenties, we were so concerned with our own immediate lives that rarely did we look ahead. That's normal for the teens and twenties—to feel we have all the time in the world and remain somewhat self-centered. We did not worry about our parents' identities or who we would become at the unimaginable ages of forty or fifty. In fact, during our twenties we wanted our parents to stay the same, so we could enjoy the stability provided by their sameness. We may have mocked them for being old-fashioned, but it was nevertheless reassuring. Then we hit our thirties, and we kept changing. Serious life decisions had to be made. And it began to dawn on most of us that there was no stable plateau. I do not know whether or not our parents found a resting point, but most of us were not to have one.

The most radical view of midlife development holds that growth continues and leads to changes in our most basic selves. This view proposes that our wishes, fears, and self-image can truly change with time. This opinion implies that there is either some continuing biological development that makes change possible or that our relationships and experiences throughout life can reshape our core selves.[5] Less radical is the idea that we can successfully battle against our pasts and develop adaptive ways of living and coping with internal conflicts. This opinion maintains that adaptive behaviors may be initially self-protective against the pain associated with our past experiences, but engaging with the world over time leads to a new sense of ourselves that brings us closer to the women we always wished to be.[6] Both beliefs support the concept that change—significant change, not just accessorizing the basic black dress—continues into adulthood.

E. Lowell Kelly collected data on three hundred engaged couples in New England between the years 1935 and 1938 and again in 1954. The average age for the women at the time of the first testing was 24.7 years old, which put them in their midforties during the follow-up. He measured attitudes, values, and vocational interests. The attitudes he tested were those toward marriage, church, child rearing, housekeeping, entertaining, and gardening. He found, for women in their middle forties, that their values and vocational interests were generally the most stable and their attitudes were the least consistent. Especially changeable were the perspectives toward marriage and raising children. This would not amaze many of us today, but the researchers in the fifties wrote, "The relative inconsistency of attitudes during the period of adulthood came as something of a surprise." They concluded that "significant changes in the human personality may continue to occur during the years of adulthood. Such changes, while neither so large nor sudden as to threaten the continuity of the self percept or impair one's day-to-day interpersonal relations are potentially of sufficient magnitude to offer a basis of fact for those who dare to hope for continued psychological growth during the adult years."[7] In a five-year follow-up to a study of midlife women, Marjorie Fiske found that some women find healthy outlets for self-expression and autonomy and their families adjust; some women compromise and, in doing so, become more assertive and bossy at home (no way to nurture their increasingly frail husbands); and some women find self-expression outside the home.[8] Psychology has come to accept adult development as a legitimate and interesting field of study, and we have also become believers, especially when we are in the middle of a transition.

Rigorous studies that examine identity changes in adult women are complicated, so, for methodological preciseness, studies examine small pieces of the personality puzzle for the generation of baby boomers and the women born a decade or so earlier. A few early longitudinal studies have actually tracked the same women, born in the late 1930s, over long periods of time. Although social and political influences differ from decade to decade, the women studied showed increased confidence, organization, and reflectiveness by their midforties.[9] These findings tell us that some changes have no relation to social forces and have more to do with maturity and normal developmental change. Social forces may have more influence on whether we get to show our new identities to the world or keep them locked up in the house, whether we are allowed to reach positions of power in corporate America or succeed exclusively in volunteer positions, and whether we gain satisfaction directly through our own activities or only through facilitating the lives of others.

IF WE LEARN NEW TRICKS, WHAT ARE THEY?

It is strange to imagine that there are aspects of our personalities that remain unavailable until the middle years. Anger is in our emotional repertoire from infancy, but assertiveness and aggression emerge and are increasingly reflected in our actions. The women I spoke with learned how to use these qualities—not against others, but in order to act for themselves. Actions allowed each woman to move ahead, conquer fears, and do more in her own life. Each woman began with small personal steps.

Fran, forty-five, divorced and remarried, left teaching art in her late thirties to begin what is now a highly successful career in corporate real estate. She talked about struggling with assertiveness and aggression, beginning years ago. When Fran was fifteen, after years of shyness and circling the fringe of groups, she finally was accepted by a popular crowd. To stay in her friends' good graces, Fran went along with just about every activity that they suggested. Finally, at the pinnacle of success in this crowd, a boy she liked confessed his affection for her. She told him that she also liked him. Thrilled, she confided this conversation to the other girls in the group, who, probably out of envy, convinced her to go back to the young man and tell him it was all a joke, humiliating him. At fifteen, in that situation, she was unable to protect herself with a normal assertive response: "Don't tell me what to do. That is an awful idea!" Instead, the next day, she told the boy it was a joke. She says that she can still see the hurt look on his face. She still feels ashamed. As Fran walked home, she became overwhelmed by aggressive thoughts directed toward her girlfriends. She wanted to kill them. Then, panicked by her intense reaction and fearful of being abandoned if she said anything to them, she turned the aggression against herself. Filled with the need to exact punishment, she got out her beloved art supplies and sliced her arm.

Years later, she understood that awful day. The aggressiveness she felt toward the girls could not be expressed in any fashion. The consequences would have been too great. She would have been alone. So she acted aggressively toward the boy and then, feeling shamed, behaved even more aggressively toward herself.

As an adult, she is more able to be assertive and aggressive when needed, but still guards against always deferring to others. "I always seem to understand other people's needs, just like I had always tried to understand my mother's needs. Of course, I didn't know any of that back then, or I might have been able to change things. I used to believe that I could tolerate anger and disappointment better than other people." Fran points to an imagined space in front of her and says, "I think I know the invisible line that others shouldn't cross. People have to respect me. This is the way I think about assertiveness. I'm not going to do their dirty work, go along, make nice, and suck it up so they are comfortable and I'm miserable. What's aggressiveness for me? Well, I'll go after a real estate deal pretty strongly. Also, if someone takes advantage of me, I'll say something to them. I'll push them back."

It took Fran a long time to understand assertiveness and aggression. "When I realized what I was doing, I got angry with everyone who I protected, then I got angry at myself for being a fool, then I realized how old the whole pattern was, and now I'm just glad I learned the lesson."

Aggressiveness and assertiveness for these women was not about beating up bullies in bars or pushing people out of line to get up front. The women went forward, when in the past, they would have talked themselves out of action before anyone else had the opportunity to discourage them.

These moves are easier in the middle years. Dimensions of personality that previously had been suppressed as incongruent with the life being led, incompatible with raising children, and in opposition to tending families, can now be liberated. When the same women graphed their level of involvement in the roles of work, partner, and mother at age twenty-seven and then again at age forty-three, they ranked involvement with the role of partner as very much the same over the years, but the role of mother peaked around the age of thirty-two and then decreased. These changes were not attributable to any one particular path, such as early childbearing versus later childbearing or an early career start versus a later career start.[10] Other research also supports this notion but found that it was particularly the women whose children were launched who showed an interesting shift toward assertiveness, mastery, and self-confidence.[11] In line with this reasoning, it has been noted that for many women in their forties, the most dramatic change in roles is the decrease in the demands of mothering, reported by 87 percent of women surveyed. These women had time and energy to release in other directions.[12] The middle years close the door on mothering, whether we have had children or whether we must face the fact that we will not. It also turns out that the emergence of assertiveness and aggressiveness is not only for mothers, who may have suppressed these qualities in favor of child rearing. A number of the women I spoke with never had children, and they were describing the emergence of exactly the same feelings of aggressiveness and assertiveness as they entered their forties.

As we age, we gain the belief that we can accomplish whatever we set out to do. Researchers suggest that with age, women become more authoritative, more effective, and less willing to trade submission for security.[13] The personality changes that occur during the middle years result from internal growth, forces that made an impact not only on our generations but on earlier ones as well, and the changes occur across ethnic groups. Middle-aged American-Irish, American-Polish, and American-Italian women showed increased activities toward realizing their own needs, and for the American-Polish and American-Italian women, there was also an increased concern with achievement and a more assertive response to their environment.[14] These same shifts are seen around the world in cultures very different from our own; women are allowed greater freedom and more power, authority, and prestige in middle age, and they no longer defer to husbands or those who are senior.[15] So, although we have been helped to express ourselves by feminism and the forces of the fifties, sixties, and seventies that taught us to protest, this aggressiveness occurs in normal female development. As women learn how to manage these new qualities with some degree of comfort, we are increasingly able to integrate these feelings into our identities, resulting in transformations toward freedom and wholeness.

AGGRESSION AND INSURGENCY

In his book *The Courage to Create*, Rollo May wrote that "creativity provokes the jealousy of the gods."[16] That image is a disturbing reminder that society protects sameness. The fear of change exists not only in you and me, but is embedded in our culture. Change requires aggression. When women initiate change, we evoke greater fear than when men make changes. To think and act for ourselves is dangerous behavior. Discarding media dictates about clothes and makeup, making decisions about our bodies, and evaluating our careers is threatening. It is not the same as a rebellious youth saying, "You can't tell me what to do!" Now, decisions reflect the thoughtful risks of adults who are willing to take responsibility for their own wishes, beliefs, and values. When we think and live creatively, we find ourselves in a struggle against the old ways. Because all societies, organizations, and families protect the way things are, creative ideas are feared as threatening to the status quo. There is good reason to fear creative ideas because they do upset the balance of things. When we say that it is fine to think, work, and feel our own experiences, that it is not bad, sick, or second-rate to value our vision, it is indeed a revolution of the first order.

All women who struggle today are artists, concerned with inner visions and images. Each is on a journey to create an authentic life rather than simply live an outdated "script," as Nan calls it. A script contains all the old roles handed to us long ago. Aggression and anger are always there when we rip up another page of the script.

It is this kind of talk that makes grown-up women dangerous to a coercive society. We have the ability to be insurgent. The women I spoke with are unsatisfied and push for newer worlds, strive to make form out of chaos. When we take action, we feel the tension between two seemingly opposite tendencies: keeping ourselves structured and together, and disrupting ourselves, allowing scattered energy and thoughts. But in spite of the danger, the lack of support, and the sense of chaos and disruption, these women kept going.

We have all heard the expression "easier said than done." After we gain a new bit of knowledge, we recognize that understanding is hard, but taking steps to change is *really hard*. Understanding and insight provide an awareness and shed light on relationships, motivations, and feelings, but insight is not action. Understanding gives us the direction in which to take action and helps bolster our confidence to make changes, but it never magically puts us at our destinations.

If it is so difficult, why bother? We keep growing because we want to hold or find the solid core of ourselves. Is it to repair the world? Yes, in part. To repair one's self? Yes. There is a phrase in Judaism, *tikkun olam*, which means "to repair the world," and a saying: "When we do an act of kindness, we recreate the world." When we repair ourselves, we have taken a step to repair the world.

In myths, many of the battles with the gods are provoked by a fight for immortality. Creativity is a yearning for immortality. We know that our personal lives are finite. One major task of adulthood is to confront and accept that fact. Yet we are also compelled to struggle and rebel against it. Creativity is part of the passion of adulthood that rebels against death by leaving something new and vital that lives beyond us. Creative growth takes fight. It is not easy to make a creation that outlasts the creator. Women have always known that about mothering—not just about the biological aspects of being a mother, but the guiding role of motherhood. When we teach children, we guide them past us. All that we have shown our children, our students, our clients, and those we mentor goes on in others beyond us. That is the real rebellion. Women are ideal as creators; biology and psychology have already given us the tools. We need the emotion to fuel action, and the emotion that allows this insurgency is anger. The anger is against injustice and inauthentic lives. Florynce Kennedy, a lawyer, advised women on political action: "You've got to rattle your cage door. You've got to let them know that you're in there, and that you want out. Make noise. Cause trouble. You may not win right away, but you'll sure have a lot more fun."[17]

NOTES

Quote in chapter title is from Joan Mills, writing about her insights: "I'd gone through life believing in the strength and competence of others; never in my own. Now, dazzled, I discovered that MY capacities were real. It was like finding a fortune in the lining of an old coat." Joan Mills, quoted in L. Clark (Ed.), (1977), *Women women women: Quips, quotes, and commentary* (New York: Drake), p. 15.

1. Nancy Chodorow, (1989), *Feminism and psychoanalytic theory* (New Haven: Yale University Press); Harriet Goldhor Lerner, (1985), *The dance of anger* (New York: Harper & Row).

2. Jean Baker Miller, (1991), The construction of anger in men and women, in J. Jordan, A. Kaplan, J. Baker Miller, I. Stiver, and J. Surrey (Eds.), *Women's growth in connection: Writings from the Stone Center* (New York: Guilford Press), pp. 181–96.

3. Ibid.

4. Lerner, *The dance of anger*, p. 1.

5. Elizabeth Auchincloss and Robert Michels, (1989), The impact of middle age on ambitions and ideals, in J. Oldham and R. Liebert (Eds.), *The middle years: New psychoanalytic perspectives* (New Haven: Yale University Press), p. 44.

6. Milton Viederman, (1989), Middle life as a period of mutative change, in Oldham and Liebert (Eds.), *The middle years*, pp. 236–37.

7. E. Lowell Kelly, (1955), Consistency of the adult personality, *American Psychologist* 10:681.

8. Marjorie Fiske, (1982), Challenge and defeat: Stability and change in adulthood, in L. Goldberger and S. Breznitz (Eds.), *Handbook of stress: Theoretical and clinical aspects* (New York: Free Press), pp. 529–43.

9. Major longitudinal studies, the Oakland Growth Study (Kelly, 1955) and the Berkeley Guidance Study at the Institute of Human Development (Helson, Mitchell, and Moane, 1984; Helson and Moane, 1987), provide support for these changes in personality. Women from Mills College, born between 1936 and 1939, have been studied several times, first as college graduates, again when they were approximately 27, again at approximately 43, and most recently at approximately age 53. These women, pre–baby boom, were young adults during the tumultuous sixties, the women's movement, and the social changes that affected marital stability, family size, and participation in the workforce. Ravenna Helson and Geraldine Moane compared the same women at age 27 and age 43 and found that at 43, the women scored higher on dominance, independence, communality, and psychological mindedness. They found that measures of traditional femininity increased from college to age 27 and then decreased. This shift was expected because measures of femininity and the feminine role tend to correlate negatively with confidence and independence, meaning that as confidence goes up, stereotypical feminine attributes go down. They found increases in coping measures on objectivity, intellectuality, concentration, and expressive coping. The women showed better coping and less defending. These findings indicate the ability to separate thoughts from feelings, to be detached from affect-laden situations, and to focus attention. The women's statements that described their feelings about life in their early forties were "having a sense of being my own person; feeling more confident; having a wider perspective; focusing on reality and meeting the needs of the day without being too emotional about them; having influence in my community or area of interest; feeling my life is moving well; feeling secure and committed; feeling a new level of productivity or effectiveness; feeling powerful; and having interest in things beyond my own family." There were also many statements reflecting concern for others and increased inner reflection, such as "feeling a new level of intimacy; having an interest in inner life; appreciating and being aware of older people; making an effort to insure that young people get their chance to develop; and discovering new parts of myself."

Helson and Moane reflect on Gutmann's works describing women becoming more "masculine," meaning aggressive and independent, qualities stereotypically attributed to men, and note that women do show more traits of confidence, independence, and assertiveness, but that this is accompanied by feelings of increased nurturance and improved relationships. The findings are more supportive of an integration of characteristics in an expanded and less defensive personality.

Florine Livson (1976) from the Institute of Human Development at the University of California, Berkeley, examined patterns of personality development in two groups of women, "traditionals" and "independents," studied as part of the Oakland Growth Study. She looked at personality evolution from adolescence to middle age in twenty-four healthy women who had been studied at intervals since they were in junior high school. Livson attempted to answer the question raised by other studies—whether the role changes that occur in middle age provide the opportunity to express other dimensions of personality previously suppressed because they were not congruent with the life being led. In other words, when we don't have to be mothers and wives in the same ways, does this role shift allow the emergence of personality traits that would have been unhelpful to the nurturing role? This question follows the line of thought that has suggested that aggressiveness and perhaps other qualities have to be suppressed in younger women because they are not compatible with the mothering role, where nurturance and softer qualities would be more desirable.

Livson found differences in personality. The independents were more autonomous than the traditional women and more in touch with their inner lives. They were not as conforming and developed skills activities rather than social activities. They gained satisfaction from developing themselves.

10. Ravenna Helson and Geraldine Moane, (1987), Personality change in women from college to midlife, *Journal of Personality and Social Psychology* 53(1):176–86.

11. David Chiriboga and Majda Thurnher, (1975), Concept of self, in M. Lowenthal, M. Thurnher, D. Chiriboga, and associates, *Four stages of life: A comparative study of men and women facing transitions* (San Francisco: Jossey-Bass). When different age groups were compared, the women between the ages of forty and fifty-five years old showed more mastery themes than the women in the younger range. The younger women appeared to lack confidence and were more troubled and dependent. In general, the women who were further along in middle age, with no children at home, showed an interesting shift toward assertiveness, mastery, and self-confidence. The noticeable difference in the postparental women in this study raises a note of caution: it reminds us that individual lives vary and the impetus for women to challenge carefully held illusions comes from many sources; this source seems to be children leaving home, but other examples could be illness, the death of a friend, or failure at work.

12. Ravenna Helson and Paul Wink, (1992), Personality change in women from the early 40s to the early 50s, *Psychology and Aging* 7(1):49. Ravenna Helson and Paul Wink studied more than one hundred women (again, the Mills College sample) who were fifty to fifty-five in 1989, the last contact. At that age, the women showed decreases in dependence and self-criticism and increases in confidence and decisiveness, traits usually associated with masculine rather than feminine stereotypes. The women reported increased comfort and stability attained through adherence to personal and social standards. They scored higher than they had previously on measures of coping through intellectuality, logical analysis, tolerance of ambiguity, and substitution. These changes suggest a growth in the capacity for systematic and impartial analysis, acceptance of complexity and uncertainty in situations, and cognitive flexibility.

Putting these changes together, we see a pattern of moving toward favorable self-concept, with gains in perseverance, achievement orientation, organization, self-esteem, self-reflection, autonomy, and the ability to engage pleasantly, considerately, and constructively with others. As the women aged, they became more organized, committed, and work oriented. They coped with life's problems more effectively and continued to increase the complexity of their interpersonal and intrapersonal perceptiveness.

13. David Gutmann, (1987), *Reclaimed powers* (New York: Basic Books). Work by Bernice Neugarten and David Gutmann, first published in 1958, is cited often, and their ideas are supported by more recent studies. They sampled a number of age groups, both men and women, using a portion of the Thematic Apperception Test. The women of interest here are the 34 women ages 40–54 and the 29 women ages 55–70. These women responded in ways that demonstrated that as women aged, after age 55 in this study, they saw themselves as changed—before 55 as sensitive to and controlled by other people's demands and pressures, and after 55 as the ones who had taken over the moral and directive qualities. In general, the trend with increasing age is to become more demanding and aggressive. Women become more self-centered instead of responsive to control by others, at least in their personalities, because actual behaviors were not measured. Neugarten and Gutmann concluded that changes in women between 40 and 70 years of age are in the direction of increased tolerance to their own aggressiveness and attention to themselves.

David Gutmann's later work, usually with people older than the women I interviewed here, argues that women do not replicate the patterns of male aging but reverse the order. He found a pattern in younger women that he described as "Passive Mastery," characterized by dependence and even deference to husbands. The pattern changes with age and becomes "Active Mastery," the belief that we can accomplish whatever we set out to do—including autonomy from and even domination over husbands. With age, Gutmann insists, women become more authoritative, more effective, and less willing to trade submission for security. This shift occurs postparenting, when women can reclaim the aggression that earlier on would have put their children at risk. When children are able to maintain their own emotional security, mothers are released to reclaim aggression, which would have been inappropriate earlier. The growth of the children frees a woman to use those energies in leadership, an idea supported by Cohler and Levy, who agree that women become more oriented toward active mastery, moving away from earlier involvement as wife, mother, and keeper of family ties and moving toward involvements beyond home and family.

Gutmann concludes that a vigorous, intense engagement with the world, even if such activity is rationalized by unrealistic ideas, will provide greater happiness for American women than a more controlled stance, however reasonable the latter might be.

14. Bertram Cohler and Morton Lieberman, (1979), Personality change across the second half of life: Findings from a study of Irish, Italian and Polish-American men and women, in D. Gelfand and A. Kutznik (Eds.), *Ethnicity and aging* (New York: Springer), pp. 227–45. Bertram Cohler and Morton Lieberman investigated ethnicity as an influence on the second half of life. Women age forty to age eighty, first- or second-generation American-Irish, American-Polish, and American-Italian, showed shifts toward increasing mastery styles, that is, actively attempting to realize one's own needs. (The reverse was found to be true for men.) And for the American-Polish and American-Italian women, there was also an increased concern with achievement and a more assertive response to their environment.

15. Karen Brodkin Sacks, (1992), New views of middle-aged women, in Virginia Kerns and Judith K. Brown (Eds.), *In her prime: A new view of middle-aged women*,

2nd ed. (Urbana and Chicago: University of Illinois Press), pp. 1–6. Sacks's ideas are supported by other cross-cultural studies in *In her prime: A new view of middle-aged women*, edited by Virginia Kerns and Judith K. Brown. The authors and editors, although they note some major differences in the display of personality between other cultures and our own, generally found heightened mobility, power and authority, and prestige in middle age; they also found that middle-aged women no longer defer to husbands or those who are senior.

There are different viewpoints as to why opportunities open up at midlife. Cultural anthropologists argue that social opportunities become more available to women as they reach the second half of life. Other researchers, working primarily in less industrialized societies, believe that the increased freedom and stature is directly related to changed sexual dynamics, either the lessened chance of bearing a child with another man or decreased sexual attractiveness to the men, making it safer to allow female authority and freedom of travel. Women who are no longer fertile have more freedom socially and geographically. It is only when women pass their peak of sexual attractiveness to men that society will allow them to have other forms of power. In many societies, women increasingly gain political power, wisdom, and healing powers. Still other views come from developmental psychologists, who argue that women change in a more liberated, autonomous direction and therefore the women themselves create new opportunities rather than simply receiving new freedoms from a more permissive society.

These advantages are contrasted with the lack of deference to and status for middle-aged women in our own society.

16. Rollo May, (1975), *The courage to create* (New York: Norton), p. 22.
17. Florynce Kennedy, quoted in Clark (Ed.), *Women women women*, p. 133.

❖ 10 ❖

"THE LONG MEANDERING FINGERS OF ICE WILL THICKEN"
Problems in Creative Living

I had already learned from more than a decade of political life that I was going to be criticized no matter what I did, so I might as well be criticized for something I wanted to do.
—Rosalynn Smith Carter

Elinor was pleased that he had called; and still more pleased that she had missed him.
—Jane Austen

No woman can call herself free who does not own and control her body.
—Margaret Sanger

There are as many impediments to creative living as there are opportunities, but certain difficulties are especially apparent in the middle years. These problems, described by the women interviewed or by individuals in therapy, warn us of the potential obstacles to growth and allow us to prepare ourselves.

Everybody has problems, so I want to go directly to the questions Which ones are yours? and How bad are they? By problems, I mean the stress, emotional reactions, and disturbances we experience because we were all brought up in imperfect families in an imperfect world where nasty things happen. Good humor helps, but it is better for each of us to know our vulnerabilities than not to know them. Knowledge is power: if we know about the trouble spots, we can try to avoid or correct them.

Clinicians who study problems in the elderly have concluded that late-onset pathology develops because we have not resolved earlier conflicts and injuries. Therefore, we continue lifestyles and coping devices that serve us poorly. Jordan Jacobowitz and Nancy Newton note that poor adult lifestyles include tendencies to avoid adult developmental tasks, repeat old patterns in a rigid manner, or restrict functioning to limited areas where we are certain to succeed.[1] By recognizing these potential problems of the later years, we are able to avoid or resolve them in midlife.

Many of the problems that interfere with creative living come from two sources: trouble reconnecting with one's self, and difficulty with the process of relinquishing outdated patterns. Much of the growth discussed depends on letting go of being young but not yet having to be old. Carolyn Heilbrun, a professor at Columbia University and mystery writer under the pseudonym of Amanda Cross, comments, "So when someone tries to compliment us who have been initiated into this special time of life by telling us we look young, we must say, 'No, not young. I am an older woman with pizazz, which is not the same thing.' "[2]

PROBLEM 1: WOMEN WHO CANNOT RELINQUISH THE OLD

We do ourselves a disservice by not mourning the past. Mourning allows us to let go. Even if we feel hurt, even if we feel empty and barren, we have to let go of the past, because if we do not, we can never reach the creativity of the future. I write about mourning because I am lousy at loss, although I admit to being pleased at my improvements. When my family left for our annual two-week vacation, we used to sneak out of the house at 5 A.M. just to avoid saying good-by to friends and relatives.

Changes and losses must be accepted intellectually, then emotionally. After we accept the change, we can adjust our self-image and our small portion of the world to match the new reality.[3] If I can learn to mourn and accept losses, so can you. If you don't, you face a desperate attempt to hang on—to what? To youth, to the kids, to eating everything you like at dinner, to pretending that you have unlimited time, or to finding a prince on a white horse. Mourning only means that we face reality, identify the losses or changes, accept whatever they mean, allow ourselves to experience genuine feelings throughout the process, and have faith that this emotional work provides a freedom of energy to reinvest in new people and new activities. Many people and ideas that we have clung to have prevented personal growth. Letting go of those inhibiting factors in our lives can encourage personality change and development.

If, after reading this far, mourning sounds like a problem for you, I suggest that you go back and reread Chapter 2, "Relinquish the Old," which describes the accessibility of the process. You may have avoided it on the first read. Take heart. We have all faced losses, and throughout these pages are stories of normal, courageous women who have changed their lives.

PROBLEM 2: WOMEN WHO RELY ON THE MANIC DEFENSE

The manic defense is an overbusyness in the external world. When individuals turn away from addressing psychological issues, we tend to think of it in terms of defense. Defense is used loosely these days; in psychology, defense refers to mechanisms, both normal and pathological, conscious and unconscious, that all of us use in order to cope with reality and at the same time protect ourselves from feeling vulnerable. One defense against unpleasant reality is a manic defense. For example, a forty-four-year-old client, aptly nicknamed Sunny, filled her life to overflowing with her children, school activities, social gatherings, and aerobics classes—way beyond the normal hectic schedule of a mother. She did not come into therapy because she was feeling uncomfortable; in fact, she rarely felt anything at all, except busy. She came in because her husband had begun to question their marriage. Sunny's first answer to the problems was to make more plans and do more things, like remodel the kitchen, but her husband objected. When she slowed down, feelings awaited her. She was forced to confront a marriage that needed repair to regain lost intimacy, her aging, her older sister's serious health problems, and children who were ready to fly. Sunny wanted to run. The sadness and emptiness was a new experience. She exemplifies the manic defense. It allowed her to avoid the fear of loss for awhile, but the price was to cut off her awareness of her inner life and psychological world. We all know people who overfill their lives with activity.

Another familiar example is the woman who remains locked into a painful marriage. This very real situation can become the focus of a manic defense. The woman pours all her energy into complaints, worries, attempts to fix, and ruminations about her marriage. The busyness gets her nowhere, but it keeps her feeling very occupied—except that it is rarely with herself that she is occupied, it is always with *him*. This situation and way of handling it contributes to a sense of stagnation.[4]

Reality is helpful. When we know ourselves, accept ourselves, value ourselves, we gain courage to act in healthy directions. Otherwise, we are trapped in the past. As much as I believe in understanding the past in order to examine the influences on our lives, we cannot live there.

If this problem sounds like your pitfall, Chapter 5, "The Psychology of Women," will help you understand these dynamics. Try to refocus on yourself. Don't ignore the people you love, but include yourself in that love and try to find the woman you misplaced—the one who does have ideas, wishes, a voice.

PROBLEM 3: WOMEN WHO FEAR ANGER AND AGGRESSION

Many women fear that aggression will damage their relationships to others. Related to that is another fear that we may not know what to do with the emerging aggressive aspects of our new midlife personalities. We have to learn to use the aspects of our personalities that emerge. Anger is an emotion, although it can frighten us when our bodies tense and prepare to fight or flee. Aggressiveness refers to action, sometimes taken as a result of anger, sometimes not. Aggression does not mean you will batter family members; it means you know what you want, say so with respect for others, and go after it. Emerging aggressiveness can become directed several ways. Some women seek opportunities for self-expression and autonomy and lower their commitments elsewhere. Many other women suffer painful inner conflict because they imagine, or realistically fear, that if they become engrossed in tasks or interests other than those that contribute to their husbands' needs, their marriages might fail. As women, we are so accustomed to responding to everyone that we often forget that others also react to us and to our emotions.

Assertiveness and self-expression may, at various times, work for or against you, but an automatic response to please others without regard to yourself, too much selflessness, and lack of self-expression have never provided women with a guarantee of living happily ever after. In fact, David Gutmann's study described and contrasted the lives of middle-aged women who were "active" with those who were "passive." The lively active women, those who used their new assertiveness to engage the world, were contrasted with the passive women, those who changed themselves rather than trying to change the world. The researchers learned that the passive women direct aggression toward themselves and become more depressed than their livelier counterparts. The passive women conform, but in doing so, see themselves as victims rather than as masters of their fate. Their energies go inward rather than outward, and they trap themselves in immobility. They may be resentful, but do not express it openly. They may not accept their fate, but cannot fight to change it. They expect that their obedience will bring rewards and are hurt when that does not happen. Unfortunately, these women become indirectly manipulative and exert power through the demands and constraints that they place on themselves and through the guilt that their deprived, depressed condition arouses in others.[5]

Chapter 9 is written to help you understand anger, aggression, and the role of these emotions and behaviors in building a creative life. Live according to the voice that guides you on the most authentic path you can find. That way, you cannot really lose, because you always have yourself. If you give yourself up, you can never win.

PROBLEM 4: WOMEN WHO FEAR CHANGE

When you change, your children, husband, lover, friends, and family will react. Just as creative work may threaten the established social order, so do your attempts to live creatively. Alterations and innovations may be discouraged by family, friends, or even religion. Change may be experienced by others as a lack of respect for the way things are or were. They react out of confusion (What in the world is she doing?) and fear (Is she going to leave me, be unavailable? Doesn't she love me anymore?). Everyone is afraid of being unloved and abandoned—not just you. Understand that people's reactions to your changes come as a result of their individual personalities, something you cannot change. Remember, others do not always want to control you. Relax and assume the least malevolent explanation until you know better.

Change happens in small steps. We imagine this sweeping flood of change taking everything in its path, but more often it is gradual, and we can pace ourselves to avoid being overwhelmed.

PROBLEM 5: WOMEN WHO BELIEVE THAT LIFE IS A REHEARSAL

Another problem that interferes with creative living is the refusal to take our own lives seriously. If we treat our life as a rehearsal and believe we get to do it "for real" next time, we will never make our lives our own. No one can give us a life—we have to make it!

I see a fifty-year-old woman in therapy named Heather. She drinks several glasses of wine almost every night and does not like the effect it has on her the next day. She also does not like her inability to control the drinking, but she has not realized that it is up to her to stop. I have had clients who drink ask me, "Aren't you going to tell me to stop?" I've had clients who injure themselves by cutting their bodies ask, "Aren't you going to take my razors?" It would take less then ten minutes after leaving my office to go downstairs, cross two streets, and purchase a razor or a bottle of alcohol. Why do we have so much trouble accepting that this life is ours? Whether it feels like a blessing or a curse, our life belongs to us and to no one else, and we must take care of it. Each of us can take care of our own lives better than anyone else ever could, especially now, in adulthood. At this time in our lives, we accept the well-earned promotion from passenger to captain.

PROBLEM 6: WOMEN WHO LIVE IN SCRIPTS WRITTEN BY OTHERS

Sometimes other people's problems shape our lives in ways that are not in our best interests at all. Claire, a lesbian who is divorced and the new owner of a unique art store, said:

I think what was important to my mother was for me to get married and live close to where she's living and to just be available to her for whatever her needs may be. She never encouraged me to continue my education. She basically encouraged me to go after [my husband] and get married, although she wasn't happy I was doing it at age eighteen. But that was her dream. I was not socialized like a lot of women to further my own self. . . . You get married and you have kids and you end up taking care of mother: that's basically what she would have wanted, and it certainly hasn't turned out that way.

Claire's mother's problems had shaped Claire's life in some very strange ways.

You see, when I was born, they gave me to an aunt and uncle to raise for the first five years. My mother had some health problems; I'm not even sure what they were. There were a lot of secrets, and they never really told me things that went on. All I ever heard from my mother, basically, was that while she carried me, the pregnancy was horrendous and delivery was horrendous. I was only told that I lived with my aunt for six months. . . . I was thirty-six at my aunt's funeral, and I made some comment about living there for six months and my cousins looked at me and said, "Claire, you were here for almost five years." And I never knew that. And they said to me, "Did you ever notice that any photograph of you as a child was always here in Connecticut with us?" I said, "Yeah, but it never occurred to me that there was anything other than maybe we were visiting."

When Claire asked her mother about this period, she was told, "I don't remember the exact details." Claire's family was unusual, but even in healthier families, there are times when our parents' needs are not good for us—are not in our best interests, but in theirs. It takes time to sort it out. As children, we want to please our parents and be loved by them. Claire tried to live the way her mother wanted; she married young, had children, bought a house nearby, and was angry all the time. It wasn't until she was close to forty years old that life became her own.[6]

If our parents are troubled, shackled by their own regrets and problems, they may demand too much from us. More subtly, they may never be aware of their demands that we fix their lives. It can all happen with no words spoken. Sometimes it is difficult even to sort out the conflicting wishes, but this time of life provides us with the maturity and confidence required to begin to think through the differences between our interests and theirs.

PROBLEM 7: WOMEN WHO CANNOT TOLERATE LONELINESS AND ISOLATION

A problem that occurs when we attempt to live creatively is the occasional sense of isolation that comes from creating. When our minds are turned inward, there is an aloneness to some aspects of the creative process that exhilarates and frightens us. This anxiety emerges because the isolation repeats our childhood fears of being alone, abandoned, or unsupported. Even the exhilaration that often accompanies being alone terrifies some of us, because we are not sure we can tolerate the accompanying anxiety. I treated one artist who, as she got closer and closer to getting rid of all the excess in her life and making it more her own, became more and more obsessed with getting pregnant. She did. It's not that the pregnancy itself was a bad idea—she is an excellent mother who cherishes every minute with her child—but the fears of becoming a productive artist had increased the desire for a baby. The baby, then, became the creative production, while making art has been delayed for an indefinite period. I know that during the first six months or so of getting into this book, when my anxiety would spike up like a fever, I would be overcome with the desire to get married. Again, there is nothing wrong with wanting to get married, but for me it came from fear created by the loneliness of writing, which made me want safety, and that translated temporarily into marriage. Luckily for me, there was no one to marry at that moment, because my wish faded as soon as my fears of this unknown book were understood.

Creative work of all kinds, including living, involves solitary time at certain stages. And we all have different levels of tolerance for being alone. I have heard many women describe how they have been consumed by the fear of being alone. Anything would be better than being alone. Yet even that fear seems to lighten in the middle years as women long for time to themselves, time to begin the reconnection with neglected elements of their personality.

PROBLEM 8: WOMEN WHO FEEL STUCK, FEEL OLD, FEEL LOST

Interviews done in 1975 found that women in the middle years were concerned about their inability to be more introspective and persevering. The research reported that the women strongly felt the need to be more imaginative. The women were vaguely discontent with the present, as if they were wondering, Where did I go wrong?[7] They were unsure of themselves and had uneasy and often conflicting characterizations of themselves. The future looked bleak to them, and they did not feel in control of their lives. They were uneasy about their own abilities and uneasy about their motivation to fulfill goals. They talked about marital dissatisfaction and feeling stressed, but had trouble explaining it.

The authors of this study found that the women had no firm identities; they had narrowed their roles and limited their activities, so the uneasiness they expressed came from anticipating future change and their need to adjust. They were looking ahead, knowingly or unknowingly; anticipating changes; and feeling uncertain of their readiness to adjust to future demands. These results have not been duplicated frequently, and certainly in the twenty years that have elapsed since those interviews, women have had many, many more options made available to them, although there are still many women today who share those feelings of discontent and vague unease.[8]

Interestingly, other research helps us find an answer to the discomfort reported by these women. Questionnaires answered by and interviews with more than two hundred married, college-educated women, aged forty-six through sixty-one years old, showed them to be generally well adjusted. The individual variables of whether or not they had an empty nest, employment level, age, socioeconomic status, level of education, whether or not they had menopausal symptoms, and their husbands' attitudes toward them were nonsignificant, indicating that the individual events that occur may not be as important as the ability to cope creatively with situations as they arise.

Creative coping skills seemed to grow out of work or volunteer activities that encouraged growth and allowed the women to test themselves in the real world in ways that increased their confidence, strong religious faith, and the ability to weather past crises, which proved to them that they could cope with problems. Lack of creative coping skills showed up in women who had not learned to depend on themselves and were overinvolved with their husbands and children. These women had not coped well with past crises and felt beaten down. The researchers concluded that self-reliance is a strength that is not encouraged in women in our society but is necessary for successful coping, and that the ability to cope with problems, not the type of problems, determines the outcome. Some of the ways of coping that the self-reliant women had learned were to expand their lives in ways that would offset the inevitable losses, to enjoy diverse roles, and to develop self reliance.[9]

PROBLEM 9: REGRET

Although mistakes, or actions taken, generate more regret in the short term, inaction, or errors of omission, produce more self-reproach in the long run. By the time we have reached midlife, we are aware that to live is to accumulate some regrets. The cliche "Don't cry over spilt milk" reminds us that regret is a popular activity. Now the question changes from How can I avoid mistakes? to How might I live so that I can keep the number and intensity of future regrets at a manageable level? To answer this question requires that we consider what people regret most and why.

The experience of regret requires a judgment, because to regret is to evaluate as well as to feel. Our anticipation of future remorse affects our present choices. For example, Lynn, a social worker in her midforties, was chronically unhappy in her eighteen-year marriage, but it was not until she looked ahead to the years she had left that she was certain she did not want to spend them with her husband. Midlife impelled her to act. Time became increasingly important. Lynn anticipated a lifetime of serious regret if she remained married, and so she left her husband. When we think about the actions taken in our lives, as Lynn did in thinking about her marriage, we evaluate the choices we actually made against "what could have been" and "what should have been." Lynn had married early because she was afraid to be alone after college. She was disturbed that she had married Joe because she saw that decision as a failure of her own courage and confidence. Most people respond like Lynn; studies show that when people reflect on their biggest regrets, they recall those things that they failed to do in their lives. When asked what they would do differently if they had another chance, middle-aged individuals answered similarly to older and younger people, giving examples of inaction, often about education. Another middle-aged group also expressed regret over things they did not do but wished they had done, and an earlier study found that women specifically said they regretted not taking more risks, not being more assertive, and not spending more time with family. Individuals regret all that was left undone in favor of other pursuits. People who spent more time on interpersonal relationships regretted lack of professional achievement. People who pursued professional success regretted not devoting enough time to family and friends, but no one regretted the time spent developing a skill or hobby.[10]

Actions involve less regret for a number of reasons. Acts more often involve a decision made at a specific choice point, like marrying early, whereas inaction more likely results from an accumulated, unfocussed pattern of not doing. More pain may be associated with actions that we regret, but there are fewer of these actions in a lifetime. The number of things we do must be smaller than the number of things we do not do, because for every action we take, there are many options we pass over. Also, we are sometimes able to mend regretted acts, so the pain can be reduced. Steps can be taken to relieve the remorse of some actions. For example, Lynn, sorry that she had married Joe, can divorce him. A client of mine returned to a store in his hometown more than twenty years later to make amends for teenage thefts. We try to overcome or undo acts that cause us shame; we apologize and attempt to get back on course. We "do" more when action is involved than when inaction is involved. Also, regrettable actions are also diminished by finding "silver linings"; for example, the marriage to Joe was a mistake, but the two children that resulted are consolation. "I learned so much" is more likely to be applied to action than to inaction. If we did not do anything, we probably did not learn much from it. Silver linings, like lessons learned, are also ways to salvage bad decisions.

When caused by inaction, the pain is not easily diminished. People are often still held in the grip of whatever caused them not to act in the first place. The ache of inaction is increased when regrets arise from an inability to conquer fear or overcome doubt, because our fears diminish over time and the further away the moment becomes, the more we believe that we could have met the challenge. The passage of time increases our confidence, but that only makes us regret inaction more.[11] We may remember why we acted in a certain way, but we have fewer satisfying explanations for inaction. When we act, for example, when we quit school, get married, or move to Wyoming, we know the consequences; they are finite. When we do not act, we wonder "what might have been" and imagine the infinite good things that would have resulted from action; events remain sadly open to perpetual recall. Regret and resentment do not improve aging. Women too often dwell in memories of what was given up. Midlife may be the final opportunity to begin the courageous acts that result in satisfaction rather than regret.

PROBLEM 10: WOMEN WHO "FAKE IT"

In treating people, I see instances where a woman has developed a "false self." Susan, a stylish, charming executive secretary married for nineteen years, came into therapy with deeply felt but vague complaints of feeling lost and sad. Among other things, it became clear that she had developed a second Susan, an overly helpful, compliant mask that she could no longer remove. This is not unusual. The false self began years before, after Susan's mother died and Susan realized that her father and the grandmother who helped raise her needed her to be docile and sweet. She complied, not wanting to be abandoned or rejected. The behavior continued throughout her life and was rewarded often, first at home and then at work, where being helpful to the vice president was highly valued. The false self, then, was her attempt to meet the expectations of others while she denied or hid her own real self. It happened out of normal desires—to feel accepted, to be loved, and to belong. Susan feared that if she behaved in new ways, she would be rejected. It is true that everyone has to learn certain roles and behaviors in order to get along in society. To a great extent this is normal; otherwise, we would have chaos. Learning to relate in ways that make us acceptable assures us a place in society. But behaviors that are not authentic and feelings that are fake, even if they make us acceptable to others, ultimately make us unacceptable to ourselves. If we do not relate with our real selves, we cannot have true intimacy, because we participate in empty relationships that remain unsatisfying. We blame ourselves because interactions are disappointing. We begin to believe that no one will ever know us, understand our feelings, or meet our needs.

This may be necessary for some people as children, and many women believe it is needed in adulthood as well. In small ways, we all "fake it": we offer false compromises and compliments, we withhold opinions, we shut up to keep the peace, and we give up aspects of ourselves here and there to make this one happy and to please that one. Middle age finds many women feeling sick of all the pretense. Others feel terribly lost. For us all, there are adjustments to be made in order to feel real again.

PROBLEM 11: WOMEN WHO BELIEVE EVERYTHING IS PERSONAL

We tend to accept responsibility for everything that goes wrong in the lives of people we love. We get caught believing that when a friend cancels lunch, when a husband is sour, when a child wasn't invited to a party or accepted at the preferred college, it has something to do with us; we said the wrong thing, we were insensitive, or we raised the child poorly. We see ourselves as involved in these events, and then we react. This is very self-centered and is reflective of illusions of control. Yes, we are important, but other people have moods and personalities and make mistakes that have nothing to do with us. Now is the time to let these things go.

PROBLEM 12: PROBLEMS FROM THE PAST—OUR MOTHERS

I am not a mother basher! I had a wonderful mother who knew how to communicate love and value better than anyone I ever met. I am also a mother, and take the role very seriously, so I always give mothers a break. But my mother was not perfect, and after being a mother for twenty-six years, I only hope that I have been "good enough" in my own mothering. I also recognize that my daughters, as wonderful as they are, will not be perfect mothers, either. There are major problems, and there are mother problems. Major problems with our mothers are way beyond the scope of this book. Basic mother problems that affect us in the middle years can be briefly addressed.

First, problems exist if your mother was not able to have a self apart from you—if she was selfless, as many of our mothers were taught to be. She never sat down at meals, ate only leftovers, did everything for Dad and us. How do we see her as distinct if she was never a clear person? She had no needs, except to be a mother. How do you become a woman with clarity, boundaries, and confidence if the most important woman in your life was lacking those qualities?

Second, problems evolve from the flip side—a mother who could not tolerate your having an existence distinct from hers. What if her needs were the only ones that counted and you had to fall in line with her needs, wishes, and desires? Hers was the only voice that counted. She was self-absorbed and did not recognize you except as she needed you to be. Mothers who were generally less empathic and were self-absorbed do not age well. They dwell on resentments and lost opportunities, which leads to envy of others and rage. They were not easy mothers when we were children, and they will be difficult even when we are adults.

Either extreme can lead to problems in our later relationships: becoming too selfless, not recognizing your abilities, or becoming vulnerable to others using you, to name a few.

Related to either end of this continuum can be another problem altogether—a mother who overanticipates the child's needs. This excessive vigilance is usually based on the mother's own fears or lack of recognition of the child's needs, and occurs when the mother continually preempts the child's attempts to do things for herself. This behavior creates an inhibition in the child because Mom jumped in too soon. Related to the mother who overanticipates a child's needs is the mother who projects (puts onto others) her feelings on the child and thereby smothers the child's own legitimate reactions. This robs the child of trust in her own experience of events.[12]

These problems are not crippling, except in the extreme, but they make it harder to feel free, to claim life as our own, to feel entitled to choose a life rather than follow a script. Having feelings, knowing what they are, tolerating emotion, valuing our own emotions and thoughts, thinking situations through so we can take action—all require emotional maturity and health. These problems may well be disturbing enough to consider therapy, because sometimes a guide is needed to help work through the tangle.

PROBLEM 13: PROBLEMS FROM THE PAST—OUR FATHERS

Fathers play a very special role in their daughter's lives. We practice being women with our fathers. Were they appalled at our emerging sexuality or aggressiveness when we were growing up? Who did they want us to become? My father's face turned a strange shade of green and he walked out of the room when, as a teenager, I strutted in my first bikini. Later, I heard him frantically whisper to my mother about the bathing suit. Luckily, she found us both amusing. But in the important matters, he was supportive; he always believed that I could be successful and encouraged me to go to college, even though he did not understand college or graduate school because he had never finished high school. Later, he was proud of my work but always worried. I think he always worried about me as his daughter; I don't know if I ever became an adult in his eyes. Also, no matter what my professional successes were, he was more interested in my being a good mother. That never changed, and there were times that I resented the narrowness of his views and his fears. All in all, I don't think we knew each other very well. It has always been amazing to me that I could love him as I did and feel his love for me, with so much left unsaid. Looking back on that time, I think he was trapped in trying to be the right kind of father—a good man, one who was decent, respectable, providing, caring. Although I believe those are essential qualities for a father, maybe he got trapped in the seriousness of the role. I still remember the few times I saw him loose and full of fun. Many of our fathers remained shadowy figures who reminded us to keep the gas tank full and not let the boys get away with anything.

Yet it is with our fathers that we gain our first sense of how to relate to a man, and from him we gain our first sense of how men will relate to us. Fathers help daughters individuate, that is, see themselves as distinct from their mothers and others. Girls look to their fathers for confirmation of their specialness and for proof of being lovable. Girls tend to idealize their fathers, but this makes it perplexing to accurately perceive our fathers' strengths and limitations. Girls are willing to deny their fathers' limitations if they feel loved, a pattern we often repeat throughout life in our relationships with men.

PROBLEM 14: WOMEN WHO HAVE PROBLEMS WITH WORK

The dynamics examined in previous problems are often displayed in work situations. Some women fear mistakes and failure to the degree that they cannot work well. In her review of work problems, Adrienne Applegarth suggests that women who cannot make mistakes have difficulty learning anything well. These women imagine that others are born with ability and cannot accept the idea that they can progress from lack of skill to skill by practice. Some women cannot tolerate the discomfort and assault to their self-esteem that come when they have to learn new skills because of this terrible fear of making mistakes. Other women are paralyzed by their strong desire to achieve, fearing they will disappoint themselves or others.[13]

Another set of work-related problems appears around handling anger and aggression. Women, because of their concern with preserving relationships, can be reluctant to express anger to bosses or subordinates. They want to be liked to an excessive degree. Unfortunately, this occasionally results in women taking on even more responsibility for other people's work. Other problems are also seen in work settings. Women who cannot take themselves seriously will have difficulty taking their work seriously. And women who cannot bear to be alone may find it impossible to think independently on the job because it makes them feel lonely and isolated.

PROBLEM 15: WOMEN WHO CANNOT ACCEPT THE POWER TO CREATE

To insure their production, all creations require that we assume some power and authority without experiencing undue guilt. Whether the creations are children, art works, teaching, novel approaches to work, or new ways to behave, some women are unable to accept this power and the resulting success. One theory suggests that if a creative act is to repair another person, the act would not raise guilt, but to create for oneself can engender guilt.[14] This theory helps to explain why a woman who feels success as a mother may not feel guilt (in this role, she acts for another person) whereas the same woman, in winning an award, can experience guilt (an award is for her creation and is her success alone).

One study reported that several artists in psychological treatment could only create in the context of sharing. The relationship with another person promoted their creativity, and their creativity collapsed without it.[15] Another study described a woman who could give her husband themes for songs but was unable to produce anything when he suggested that she create songs on her own, because her inspiration came only if the song was to be his. On examining this block in treatment, it was found that the client's father was an amputee; she had helped him in many ways, including driving; and he had been proud of her. She created in order to repair her father's missing limb. Her creations were prostheses. She could not allow personal initiative in which she, not the other person, would be the possessor of the production. When creation is not possible without someone else to share it, the art process shifts into someone else's hands. Whether the fear of creation comes from a general fear of being out of control, fear of being different, fear of aloneness, or fear of the selfishness in attending to ourselves, we will suffer inhibition in the creative aspects of living.[16]

It may reassure us to remember that creativity's deepest impulse, its living strength, is essentially linked to freedom. The creative act whose end is the restoration of our own integrity will be more beneficial to us. But all creative acts bring us closer to our own integrity by giving us a psychic completeness and allowing us to overcome gaps and deficiencies in our past, in our upbringing, and in our maturation. Creative acts can heal, by our own means, damage caused by others.

OTHER PROBLEMS

I have not touched on the severe problems of sexual and physical exploitation, families in which drugs and alcohol were abused, parents who were violently destructive, and other appalling experiences. I have not forgotten them. Rarely a day goes by when I am not talking about the terrible results of these problems with men and women, but this is not the place for them. A cursory glance at problems of abuse is an insult; it diminishes the complexity involved in understanding them and ignores the work involved in healing them. So I knowingly sidestep the more severe problems. Some of the women interviewed did come from very disturbed families; most did not. Creative living does not require a fantastic family, but a good beginning helps. All families have legacies, good and bad, but in the middle years, if life is to remain our own, we must make headway on any problems that have resurfaced or have been ignored until this time.

Julia Cameron, in *The Artist's Way: A Spiritual Path to Higher Creativity*, recalls a wonderful, old, hostile question: "But do you know how old I will be by the time I learn to really play the piano/act/paint/write a decent play? Yes—the same age you will be if you don't. So let's start."[17]

NOTES

Quote in chapter title is from "The Impasse" in Joyce Carol Oates, (1975), *The fabulous beasts* (Baton Rouge: Louisiana State University Press), p. 6.

1. Jordan Jacobowitz and Nancy Newton, (1990), Time, context, and character: A life-span view of psychopathology during the second half of life, in R. Nemiroff and C. Colarusso (Eds.), *New dimensions in adult development* (New York: Basic Books), pp. 310–11.

2. Carolyn Heilbrun, (1991, Summer), Naming a new rite of passage, *Smith Alumnae Quarterly*, pp. 26–28.

3. Milton Viederman, (1988), Personality change through life experience: Two creative types of response to object loss, in D. Dietrich and P. Shabad (Eds.), *The problem of loss and mourning: Psychoanalytic perspectives* (New York: International Universities Press), pp. 187–212.

4. Arnold Modell, (1989), Object relations theory: Psychic aliveness in the middle years, in J. Oldham and R. Liebert (Eds.), *The middle years: New psychoanalytic perspectives* (New Haven: Yale University Press), pp. 17–26.

5. David Gutmann, (1987), *Reclaimed powers* (New York: Basic Books).

6. Claire wants her story dedicated to Aunt Kitty.

7. Marjorie Fiske Lowenthal, Majda Thurnher, and David Chiriboga, (1975), *Four stages of life* (San Francisco: Jossey-Bass), p. 131.

8. Lowenthal, Thurnher, and Chiriboga, *Four stages of life.*

9. Sionag Black and Clara Hill, (1984), The psychological well-being of women in their middle years, *Psychology of Women Quarterly* 8:282–92.

10. Thomas Gilovich and Victoria Husted Medvec, (1995), The experience of regret: What, when and why, *Psychological Review* 102(2):379–95.

11. Ibid.

12. Nancy Chodorow, (1989), *Feminism and psychoanalytic theory* (New Haven: Yale University Press).

13. Adrienne Applegarth, (1986), Women and work, in T. Bernay and D. Cantor (Eds.), *The psychology of today's woman: New psychoanalytic visions* (New York: The Analytic Press), pp. 214–22.

14. Janine Chasseguet-Smirgel, (1984), Thoughts on the concept of reparation and the hierarchy of creative acts, *International Review of Psychoanalysis* 11:399–409.

15. Sanford Weisblatt, (1977), The creativity of Sylvia Plath's Ariel period: Toward origins and meanings, *The Annual of Psychoanalysis* 5:379–404. Weisblatt lists factors suggested by others that may influence the productivity or quality of an artist's work:

1. The presence of a secret sharing in which the relationship with another person promotes creativity. The creativity collapses without the secret sharing.

2. The impact of death and grief promotes creativity as an undoing, penance, or commemoration of impending reunion.

3. The anticipation of one's death encourages creativity as an attempt to stave it off.

4. Creativity is a depression-inspired effort to use the created object as a replacement for a part of one's self.

These factors amplify the idea in Chapter 4 that a creation serves to replace a person or a part of one's self and supports the finding that many creative people have lost a loved one in childhood and that loss is temporarily healed by artistic production. The creation stands in fantasy for that lost person, ideal, or illusion.

16. Chasseguet-Smirgel, Reparation and hierarchy of creative acts.

17. Julia Cameron, (1992), *The artist's way: A spiritual path to higher creativity* (New York: Tarcher/Perigee), p. 30.

❖ ❖ ❖

PART III
REFOCUS THE FUTURE

In the world to come, they will not ask us,
"Why were you not Mother Teresa?"
They will ask, "Why were you not Linda
(Susan, Nancy, Carol, Jen . . .)?"

STARTING OUT

Transitions are bridges—beginning here and ending there. No one lives on a bridge; we cross them, often with a combination of fear and exhilaration.

As teenagers in New Jersey, my friends and I used to picnic on the rocks directly underneath the George Washington Bridge. The bridge stretched over me right into Manhattan. Everything familiar was on my side of the bridge. All my dreams were on the other. This kind of experience marks the beginning of a transition. Change begins with this kind of an encounter with something new—an idea or dream, a place, or an aspect of ourselves, just revealed.

Transition has become an increasingly popular term and reflects the increased attention being paid to adulthood as a dynamic rather than a static period of life, a period with different phases and tasks. The tasks of a developmental transition are

to terminate a time in one's life: to accept the losses the termination entails; to review and evaluate the past; to decide which aspects of the past to keep and which to reject; and to consider one's wishes and possibilities for the future. One is suspended between past and future and struggling to overcome the gap that separates them. Much from the past is given up—separated from, cut out of one's life, rejected in anger, renounced in sadness or grief. And there is much that can be used as a basis for the future. Changes must be attempted in both self and world.[1]

The shared feature of all transitions is this bridgelike quality of being between an old home and a new one, headed toward the new but faced with the necessity of doing the work that increases the chance of a safe arrival. Sometimes, we don't even know what the work is—only that we experience discomfort and want to understand more about ourselves. This is when we feel the mourning and loss.

MIDAIR

We are seated at the circus. In the center ring above our heads, dressed in a sparkle-white costume, is the trapeze artist. Her partner hands her the bar. She holds it, swings from her perch into the center of the tent, releases her hold—we gasp!—and she grabs the second bar that carries her safely to another perch above. We breathe. There was a fragment of a moment when she was in midair alone. Transitions include that moment, but in real life, the time in midair, when we hold on to nothing, can last for weeks or months.

ARRIVING HOME

I used to sit in the back seat of my father's Chevy (it was always a Chevy) as he drove home from the two-week winter vacation in Florida (it was always Florida). The last leg of the three-day trip (it was always . . .) was the New Jersey Turnpike, and when we reached Exit 9, my mother would point it out, and I would burst into my off-key rendition of "Be it ever so humble, there's no place like home!" Transitions bring us to that moment.

When psychological transitions are successful, we have let go of the old and we have walked, flown, driven—or crawled—through a process of mourning that can establish us in a new, consolidated life with more freedom and clarity of identity.

MARGARET'S DREAM

Margaret provides us with a wonderful example of a transition and the dream she had in the midst of it. Margaret had come into therapy when she was forty-eight. She was tall, had gorgeous skin, and was unusually honest—with herself and others—so working with her was a pleasure from the start. She told me that she wanted to make some changes in order to feel less depressed and more in control of her own life. She was happily married for the second time but otherwise dissatisfied. Work as a self-employed book editor did not feel like her own, and her drinking controlled her more than she ruled the red wine. Her real love was collecting and making quilts, a craft about which she was passionate and knowledgeable.

Margaret had been in therapy a couple of other times during her adulthood but, as she described the treatment, it seemed to me that she had spent entirely too much time either complying with or fighting other people's rules. No wonder she didn't feel like she owned her life. Both conforming and rebelling shifted the focus away from her and onto others. Unfortunately, when she made the rules, she fought them with equal vigor.

One central issue at this time was, "It's time to take yourself seriously." She exercised little control over her life and treated it as though it belonged to somebody else.

Margaret's life looked better to others than it felt to her. She appeared to take herself seriously and worked hard, but never outgrew criticisms that hammered her: "You must be productive—do what you say you will do." Of course, it was never enough. The other particularly stunting criticism was, "Don't be full of yourself," which had for years kept her passive and deferential outwardly but stubborn and willful in secret. Her life had been reactive to these now conscious commands, so Margaret entered a serious struggle to reclaim her life—and she was winning. It was time to begin to create.

She had been in therapy approximately fifteen months when she went to an alumni meeting for her beloved college. She roomed with an old acquaintance, Anne, and came back very impressed. In her friend, Margaret saw a gracious woman who had made peace with herself, accepted the necessary accommodations to make her married life successful—having no children and giving up a career—and Anne still felt that she had made a good bargain. It was not that Margaret admired the sacrifices, or even agreed with them. She admired Anne's attitude, which conveyed the feeling that she had done well, had made conscious choices and was pleased with her decisions. Anne was a participant in life, and this attitude made an impact.

Margaret turned fifty shortly afterward and felt good. Fifty years old, she said, made her an adult. Three weeks postbirthday she reported the following dream, which described her transition.

I dreamed that I was in a country that wasn't a desert but it was brown, the ground, like there had been a drought. I was going to be there nine months and would go home in the summer. Wouldn't Dan [her husband] be surprised that I was away, but I knew that it was okay with him. Then I realized that I needed shoes, so a bunch of us hopped into a car that was there for us, and we drove into the village. I remember thinking that I wished I had brought my camera. The village was beautiful. There were living areas with streets and homes and there were shops. There were so many colors. I was looking in the shops for fabrics and textiles. I found all kinds of wonderful things, but I decided not to buy the fabrics right away because I was going to visit that country for a while and had plenty of time to enjoy the materials and choose my favorites. My mother was there with me at that point in the dream, and she became impatient and wanted me to get on with buying them, already.

I went back into the room where I was going to stay and opened my suitcase. I had loads of shoes and I realized that I didn't have to take all of them back home with me when I left because I had extras. I also had my camera.

As Margaret thought about the dream in an uncensored way, she said that the shoes were a metaphor for the basic necessities of life. At first, she had none and then she had more than enough, even extras. The length of her stay, nine months, made her immediately think of pregnancy and creative production. The desert is an image of transition—wandering in a dry land, looking for home. The desert also captures the endless, barren feelings that accompany change—a nowhere place. People, ideas, and dreams have been left behind, but new ones have not yet replaced them—like the midair moment of the trapeze artist.

The dream illustrates the experience of a transition nearing its end. When we come home, after we have changed, even our homes are new places, because these regions are now combinations of thoughts and ideas we had not previously put together.

This last section of the book reflects on the final stages of midlife change, the work and rewards. The women describe their turning points, and I examine the courage necessary to take risks and become vulnerable. We see how the changes they made internally are displayed in the world, often in work, and they tell us about their dreams and achievements.

NOTE

1. Daniel Levinson, (1978), *The seasons of a man's life* (New York: Alfred A. Knopf), p. 51.

❖ 11 ❖

"LIFE SHRINKS OR EXPANDS IN PROPORTION TO ONE'S COURAGE"
Finding Courage

I cannot and will not cut my conscience to fit this year's fashion, even though I long ago came to the conclusion that I was not a political person and could have no comfortable place in any political group.
—Lillian Hellman, excerpt from a letter she wrote to the House Committee on Un-American Activities

Courage is the price that Life exacts for granting peace.
—Amelia Earhart

It isn't for the moment you are stuck that you need courage, but for the long uphill climb back to sanity, faith and security.
—Anne Morrow Lindbergh

It is better to die on your feet than to live on your knees.
—Delores Ibarruri (known as La Passionaria)

Let me listen to me and not to them.
—Gertrude Stein

Courage is essential at midlife because it allows us to take the risks necessary to refocus our lives. In *The Wizard of Oz*, Dorothy reassures the Scarecrow after her dog, Toto, sniffs and growls at him.

"Oh, I'm not afraid," replied the Scarecrow; "he can't hurt the straw. . . . I'll tell you a secret," he continued, as he walked along; "there is only one thing in the world I am afraid of."

"What is that?" asked Dorothy; "the Munchkin farmer who made you?"

"No," answered the Scarecrow; "it's a lighted match."[1]

In each of our lives, we fear the lighted matches, and rarely can we extinguish them. We are vulnerable to fear but want to go on anyway. And we can. That is why courage is essential. If taking thoughtful risks is the road to creative change, then the vehicle is courage. We can rely on courage to carry us during the process. Change takes time; we do not create ourselves in a single act, but instead we make humble decisions every day that accumulate to form our individual lives. As we face the issues presented on previous pages, courage allows us to mourn, to find ourselves, to accept ourselves and others, to trust our feelings and decisions, and to stay with the process as we move closer to our authentic selves. Even the people we love have a difficult time if we change. They do not applaud us. They may be worried that we will change too much or leave them. Yet the process continues, because there is some push toward the sunlight, as with the Little Engine that Could or the surprising morning glories from my childhood, which shoved their way through our black asphalt backyard to bloom year after year.

WHERE DO WE FIND COURAGE?

Years ago I turned to my imagination and created my own personal warrior-guide. She is an old lady sitting on a front porch in a rocking chair. This is all fantasy, of course. My old lady has never existed in the world I know; I think she is the missing piece of my own mother. In my fantasy, it is a glorious day. I sit on broad porch steps and spill out my problems. She asks, "Do you want to be filled with regret when you are sitting in this rocking chair? What do you want to see when you look back? Who do you want to be able to say that you have been?" We all find ways to hang on to whatever courage is inside. My old lady links me to determination and helps fight the fears.

We can all do this—reach inside ourselves for encouragement or support. To store up courage inside, we gather outside support from friends, family, books, classes, or professionals. Women excel at mutual relationships, and midlife is the ideal time to cultivate healthy, supportive groups. People who care about us provide excellent protection against insecurity. They help us to remember to take care of ourselves and to lighten up and let the unimportant matters drift away, they validate our beliefs and feelings, and they share many similar experiences.

When mutually empathic and supportive relationships are gone, women move into isolation and feel immobilized. The empowerment that comes from healthy relationships is lost, and we find it difficult to act in our own best interest. Talking and sharing feelings, the strategies that women seem to be particularly good at, work well in the early stages of defining problems and in situations where we actually have little control. When we talk to others who are able to listen to us, we organize our ideas and gain clarity in our beliefs. The more masculine strategy of taking action to solve the problem works well once we have direction and in situations where change is possible.

Help seeking is scorned in this country, yet it is particularly effective for women to mobilize us to action. When we are connected, whether to a person, belief, or goal, we are energized because we are a part of something larger than ourselves. It feels good to be able to both give and take. Vital relationships supplement or replace tired ones. We need connections to avoid depletion, and strong relationships in one area of life help to overcome deprivation in another.[2]

COURAGE IS A COLLECTION OF SMALL ACTS

Every life requires some courage. Some lives necessitate a great deal. S. Josephine Baker, M.D., believed in her work, and over her lifetime her devotion to medicine propelled her into areas she had never anticipated and kept her going. She noted, years later, that perhaps her ambition was at first motivated by trying to make it up to her father for being born a girl. Her ambition became unshakable when a younger brother, and then her father, died of typhoid when she was just sixteen. She considered herself "elected." Dr. Baker (1873–1945), whose mother had been a member of the first class of Vassar, left home to become a physician only to find that the over-whelming prejudice that existed prevented her from earning a living as a doctor. Friendship with other women and the opportunities afforded by living in New York helped her endure the prejudice. She earned some money practicing as a doctor, but her major income was secured through work in public health as a medical inspector and, later, through teaching at New York University. The work she did in public health altered her path. She authored five books about children and more than fifty articles on child hygiene, child welfare, and public health. She was an important figure in the development of public health and child welfare.

Then, at age forty-one, life picked up greater speed. She wrote,

Up to 1914 [age forty-one], I think I could conscientiously have testified on oath that, in my opinion, I was leading a fairly active life. . . . Everything started whirling at once that year: why I do not know. Suffrage for instance. . . . In the spring of 1914 I received a letter from the Philadelphia College of Physicians asking me to read a paper before them. . . . I assumed that the Philadelphia College of Physicians was about the same as the New York Academy of Medicine, an institution with which I have had many contacts. . . . [T]he members' faces froze into paralytic astonishment as I passed.[3]

She found out that it was the first time a woman had been allowed to enter the premises. That was more than fifty years after women had begun to practice medicine in America, and "periodicals of all kinds had been talking about the New Woman for thirty years."

The next year she began to lecture at Bellevue and recalled,

Every lecture I gave at Bellevue, *from 1915 through to 1930*, was clapped in and clapped out . . . not the spontaneous burst of real applause that can sound so heart-warming, but instead the flat, contemptuous whacking rhythms with which the crowd at a baseball game walks an unpopular player in from the outfield. [Italics mine]

By that time I was in the middle of the suffrage fight. I have explained that I did not start out as a feminist at all. But it was impossible to resist the psychological suction which gradually drew you into active participation in the great struggle to get political recognition of the fact that women are as much human beings as men are. Fundamentally that was what we were all after.[4]

Dr. Baker continued for fifteen years with the sounds of contemptuous clapping and endless prejudice. We see all the elements of women's courage in her story. Her endeavors were made day-to-day, not in one spectacular display. Dr. Baker's story sounds more extraordinary because her adulthood is condensed into three hundred words. She faced hostility from others. Her bravery came in her ability to follow a belief in spite of the devaluation coming from her colleagues. Yet she is not very different from Susan, who investigated every opportunity for the disabled so that her handicapped child had a chance. Ellen nursed her young husband for ten years until his death. Nancy fought to get a library built so reading was free and available to everyone. Sara battled her own depression so that her family had a better upbringing than she had had. Gwendolyn worked two jobs and paid the mortgage on time every month for twenty years. These women showed fortitude. We find courage when we come up against our values and have to act on our beliefs, great or small. Does it take being a doctor or an artist to live fully? All the women I talked to told me stories that demonstrated courage.

COURAGE CREATES OPPORTUNITIES

Emma, forty-two, showed courage when faced with a terrible situation. She not only dealt with it, but discovered new strengths and opportunities in the crisis. Emma told her story in a very matter-of-fact tone of voice, which made it hard to know whether to laugh or cry. Her husband, Gene, a business executive, had been married before and had two sons in college; together, they had one young daughter. Emma and Gene lived a high life-style filled with money, position, and social standing. She worked a little bit from home but did not consider herself a career woman.

She looks back and says,

My story is not that uncommon these days—all caused by a single event—my husband is an alcoholic. He needed to go into the hospital, which he did. However, [after he entered the hospital], I found out that the life we were leading was a total lie. We were living in a penthouse in San Francisco. He took care of finances. There were bills that he was hiding. We were incredibly in debt. Tuition for his sons' schools hadn't been paid. We had been married about five years at the time. I got a lot of bad news. I was home trying to hold body and soul together. My family never really liked my husband. It was very difficult for them to be supportive. However, my friends were terrific.

We were evicted. I had to take [our daughter] Kim out of private school. It seemed best to go to the suburbs, where she could get a good education and I could try to clean up this mess. We had no medical coverage. I needed to find a job, "like yesterday." I had been doing some marketing from home. I needed medical benefits. I applied for a job at Marin Hospital and was pretty aggressive. It was total desperation. That is what spurred the whole thing on.

Emma viewed her motivation as coming from sheer urgency.

"Would I have evolved this way? I think not. . . . I've learned I can rise to any occasion. I'm a survivor. I've been tested. The kids have learned to be survivors. The lifestyle I thought I was going to live is not the lifestyle I will be living."

In Emma's response to her lost dreams, her creative courage became most evident.

I think I began to see the other possibilities. I gained a perspective that is healthier. I have acquaintances that are into acquiring physical goods rather than doing other things that are more rewarding, reading a good book. How many shoes do you need? . . . I think that has made me more open to people from all walks of life. I think I was less inclined to listen to someone's tale, to put myself into someone's shoes. I can listen more openly instead of, So what, that doesn't affect me. I'm more multifaceted in my capabilities than I gave myself credit for. I forced myself to try things under the guise of economic threat—to do things that I wouldn't ordinarily do.

Emma told me an extraordinary story of getting an evening job, after her regular work, as the Easter Bunny at her former golf club, where her parents and friends still had memberships. There, she passed out eggs to the children and told them stories.

"As I left work, I am memorizing this story that I wrote for the Club. I get into the costume as I am driving, got to the Club and put on four of these performances during the Easter season, incognito. We needed money."

She was completely disguised in a giant purple bunny outfit. Instead of the embarrassment that many other people would have felt, Emma turned financial need into an opportunity. She was proud of meeting these challenges creatively rather than bemoaning the lost luncheons and social status.

"I think perspective changes with age naturally. I think some [of my] friends will arrive at similar points without going through all this. But would they arrive if they hadn't stood up with me? They had to take a look at themselves." Emma was lucky to have good friends. It is natural to form and maintain lasting and positive relationships that contain an enduring sense of care and concern for each other's welfare.[5] Through these friendships we learn from others' experiences. As Emma changed, some of her friends were also changed.

Emma and the other women I spoke with evaluated their courage very modestly. Emma said, "I don't see it as courageous. I see it as doing what is necessary. I didn't see choices. They were real limited." Another said, "But it doesn't seem like courage as such because the risk of what's behind you is worse." A third woman said, "It's what I have to do, and it's not difficult for me anymore. It was. It was very painful."

The women all made lemonade out of lemons. That was a choice, whether they saw it or not, and a choice made not out of blindness or lack of alternatives. Emma could have moved home. Her parents wanted her to leave Gene and would have supported her. She had thought about separating but did not want Gene's sons to deal with his alcohol problems alone, did not want to be a single mother, and "was not a quitter." She stayed.

The women I spoke with failed to consider their actions as courageous because ordinary daily events were involved—not life-and-death decisions. The moment they realized that they could try again, or pick themselves up off the floor if they fell, they began to undervalue the courage that is required for vulnerable acts.

COURAGE AND RISK

Courage helps us to take chances, because each time we take a risk, we are exposed to the unknown. The women I spoke with were not always eager to charge forward. Some women took risks because they had "nothing left to lose" or, as Isabelle said, "The alligator behind is worse than the one ahead." When we choose between bad and awful, when we are desperate and our backs are to the sea, we can go for broke. But even then, we learn that we can endure. Life does not wait for us to be ready for a challenge. When we face trouble and survive, if we give ourselves credit, confidence and esteem are enhanced. If we minimize our actions or attribute our successes to luck, we gain nothing.

The women I interviewed and the women I have worked with in therapy did not start out with high self-esteem. Quite the opposite; many lacked confidence and were intimidated by feelings of insecurity. For them, courage included an acceptance of their vulnerabilities and respect for personal limitations as well as for strengths.

Certainly, we are in a better position to take chances when our self-esteem is secure. Then, we know that we can emotionally survive the outcome. This may explain why women with healthy self-esteem are able to accept risks as a valuable aspect of life.

A New Definition of Courage

The women shared certain internal qualities that anchored them. Each accepted her view of events as valid, held on to her integrity, and was willing to be vulnerable. They learned that vulnerability can come from strength, not weakness. Even when outside events, such as a husband's illness, divorce, monetary need, or job problems, set change in motion, each woman chose her response. How each woman changed and whether she would change in healthy ways was still up to her. Even when circumstances are forced on us, we have choices about our response. We cannot control the world or even our small part of it, but we can take initiative and determine our response and our reply to people and events.

Courage does not mean the absence of fear. Emma said candidly, "I was terrified." She was afraid that she would raise her child alone, in poverty. Others had different fears. Ann was terrified of emotion; she had no fear of the physical world. She is strong and comfortable out of doors, but terrified at being abandoned in relationships. Isabelle was afraid that she would live on the surface rather than in the depths if she did not make a change. Megan was afraid to trust others, especially men. Melanie was afraid of being alone. One was afraid of taking risks; another was afraid that she was not strong enough to meet the challenges. Laura was afraid that she was not good enough. The fears that have to be acknowledged and respected are as many as the women there are.

These women were not brave because they never felt fear; they were brave because they overcame fear. Courage is not the reckless bravado of war movies. Courage is the ability to act in times of fear. Laura knew that when she said, "Very recently, I've begun to see myself as courageous in an odd way."

The women were motivated to persevere by their commitments, best judgments, and values grounded in the center of their beings. Research suggests that our ability to continue new behaviors depends not only on the benefits we expect but also on our sense of mastery—whether we initially believe that we can succeed. Lack of confidence, more than actual failure, is a major cause of giving up.[6]

I do not know how many women would have made the same decisions Emma made. I have no idea how many of us could have survived the prejudice and contempt that S. Josephine Baker endured. I do not know what I would have done in either situation, and it does not matter. What is important is that each woman acted in ways that were consistent with her beliefs. Some beliefs lie dormant and are uncovered only when we face our internal and external worlds. Emma is unusual because she used a terrible situation to try new behaviors. These were behaviors that she never would have attempted without some outside reason that allowed her to discard all the old socially acceptable ways of doing things and try something new. She broke out of the old mold and found a better way. And in the process, she widened her world, learned more about herself and others, and gained trust and confidence in her ability to manage life.

Women's courage requires a new definition. Psychologist Judith Jordan suggests that courage, "unlike macho defiance of fear, is the capacity to act meaningfully and with integrity in the face of acknowledged vulnerability. There is no real courage where fear and vulnerability are denied."[7] Courage then, is the action that comes with our full awareness of risk, tempered by self-reflection and confidence. This form of courage becomes most apparent in contrast to the alternative—a life of stagnant complacency or helplessness in which challenges are seen and felt but avoided. Proving that they have courage was never the goal for these women. For them, courage is what it takes to get to the goal. We all show courage when we overcome fear, trust ourselves, and believe in the goal we are aiming toward.

And where is the creativity? Courage is necessary for the expression of oneself, and that expression, in whatever form, is creative. Action taken from the center of us is the foundation for a refocussed life. "If you do not express your own original ideas, if you do not listen to your own being, you will have betrayed yourself. Also you will have betrayed our community in failing to make your contribution to the whole."[8]

NOTES

Quote in chapter title is from Anais Nin, quoted in Julia Cameron, (1992), *The artist's way: A spiritual path to higher creativity* (New York: Bantam), p. 156.

1. L. Frank Baum, (1979), *The wizard of Oz* (New York: Ballantine Books), p. 30, originally published in 1900.

2. Judith Jordan, (1992), Relational resilience, Work in Progress, No. 57 (Wellesley, MA: Stone Center Working Paper Series).

3. S. Josephine Baker, (1992), Fighting for life, in J. K. Conway (Ed.), *Written by herself* (New York: Vintage Books), p. 165.

4. Ibid.

5. Roy Baumeister and Mark R. Leary, (1995), The need to belong: Desire for interpersonal attachments as a fundamental human motivation, *Psychological Bulletin* 117(3):497–529.

6. National Advisory Mental Health Council, (1995, October), Basic behavioral science research for mental health: A national investment, emotion and motivation, Rockville, MD, *American Psychologist* 50(10):844.

7. Judith Jordan, (1990), Courage in connection: Conflict, compassion, creativity, Work in Progress, No. 45 (Wellesley, MA: Stone Center Working Paper Series), p. 2.

8. Rollo May, (1975), *The courage to create* (New York: Norton), p. 3.

"DON'T DREAM IT, BE IT"
Turning Points

I love my husband very, very much, but he didn't ask me when he ran for mayor and he didn't consult me about running for governor. It would be nice to be asked.

. . . You know, I've been my mother's daughter, my father's daughter, the wife of my husband, the mother of my six children, and a grandmother to my eleven grandchildren, but I have never been me. But I am now because I went away. I am a changed woman.

—Angelina Alioto, wife of a California politician, after disappearing for eighteen days

When things go wrong, don't go with them.
   —Anonymous

I didn't know that I could leave.
   —Client, age forty-nine

I didn't know that I could leave.
   —Client, age thirty-nine

I didn't know that I could leave.
   —Client, age twenty-seven

The change process often begins with moments of illumination and insight when we bump into ourselves or others and are redirected by the encounter. When women told me about the exciting changes they made in their lives, my question was, "How did you begin?"

Each one of us brings to the turning points in life our personality, history, accumulation of experience, and myriad influences. There is much we have in common, but because of our idiosyncrasies, the processes of mourning our losses and the reconnection to ourselves is entirely personal. Therefore, in the final steps to refocussing our futures, among us we find similar underlying dynamics but one-of-a-kind moments when we summon our courage and take a step that turns us onto a different path. Remember, the Skin Horse cautioned the Velveteen Rabbit on becoming real, "It doesn't often happen to people who break easily, or have sharp edges, or who have to be carefully kept."[1]

ENCOUNTER

All turning points first require an encounter with ourselves and the world around us. Encounters with ourselves inform us about what is inside, just as encounters with the world teach us about the outside. In this way, confrontations give us more knowledge of who we are and what we can do, contributing to our confidence. Our perspective of our own response is enlarged, and we hold a broader picture of ourselves than previously. As we continue to encounter what we see and feel, we become increasingly secure in our abilities to meet new situations effectively. On my most recent vacation with my daughters, we swung in harnesses from tree to tree eighty feet above ground. I am afraid of heights. I have no desire to repeat the experience, but it was a victory for me. Successful encounters challenge us but do not defeat us, because challenge produces a level of frustration that is not great enough to make us want to give up but demands an effort. When we succeed, even in swinging from tree to tree, we feel proud to be able to master another bit of life.

To encounter is to keep the appointment; first we encounter, and then we engage. To engage is to enter a covenant with, a commitment to, or even a collision with these new internal and external forces.

ENGAGEMENT

Women, having been brought up to value connectedness, are skilled at engagement. We see this skill in the myriad of commitments made to school, church, friends, and the family, but it proves difficult for women to get involved in activities outside the socially acceptable range. My premise, though, is that the ability to engage can be expanded; new forms of involvement are possible because we can use our newfound confidence, courage, and aggressiveness.

Opportunities to engage are found with each encounter. We take part in life moment to moment, from the most humble tasks to the most lofty, so it becomes important to engage mindfully, not absently. Eleanor Roosevelt provides a notable example of a woman who, by the nature of her position rather than her inherent disposition, increasingly encountered and engaged her world. The choices she made at critical junctures shaped her life. In her inspiring autobiographies, we learn that her fears and risks were remarkably similar to those of every woman.

Eleanor Roosevelt was born in 1884 and married at twenty-one years old in 1905. She describes herself at twenty-four years old, in her new home, as crying bitterly in front of her confused young husband, Franklin. When he asked her what was wrong, she told him that she did not like to "live in a house which was not in any way mine, one that I had done nothing about and which did not represent the way I wanted to live."[2] Many years later, reflecting on this incident, Eleanor saw the truth in those words and believed that she was absorbing the desires of those around her rather than creating initiatives of her own.

She reflects in a remarkably forthright manner on her transcendence from a timid young woman to a person of secure and independent judgment. As a young woman, she was so attuned to others and eager to please that she had no voice of her own. She remembers the first inkling of the woman she was to become when the family moved to Albany in 1910 because Franklin was elected a state senator. "I had to stand on my own feet now and I wanted to be independent. I was beginning to realize that something in me craved to be an individual." In 1913, they moved to Washington, D.C., and her last child was born in 1916. She noted that "for ten years I was always just getting over having a baby or about to have one."[3] Eleanor was occupied with caring for others, listening to others, and obeying others. Her mother-in-law had ruled her life for years, but Eleanor finally realized, "I looked at everything from the point of view of what I ought to do, rarely from a standpoint of what I wanted to do. There were times when I almost forgot that there was such a thing as wanting anything."[4]

Five years later, at age thirty-one, she "was beginning to acquire considerable independence again because my husband's duties made it impossible for him to travel with us at all times." She began to encounter people and events on her own, using her eyes, not anyone else's vision. At thirty-three years old, she voiced her difference of opinion about serving in the war. "This was my first really outspoken declaration against the accepted standards of the surroundings in which I had spent my childhood, and marked the fact that either my husband or an increasing ability to think for myself was changing my point of view."[5] She began to voice opinions that grew from her own ideas and thoughts.

The armistice ending the war was signed in 1918. The war changed many lives and attitudes. Old patterns had been shattered and were never going to be rebuilt in quite the same way. Eleanor Roosevelt, like many women, had responded to emergencies and crises. She wrote that she had "gained a sense of values."[6] Once she began responding out of her own firmly held beliefs, she could separate important matters from nonessentials, and she would no longer be as easily bullied or coerced by others.

Her values had broadened beyond family to embrace social issues that reflected her priorities. She was losing patience for unimportant commitments. During the next couple of years, Eleanor had her first real contact with the women's suffrage movement. "I became a much more ardent citizen and feminist than anyone about me in the intermediate years would have dreamed possible."[7] The changes were just beginning. In 1920, she was thirty-six years old and wrote that the war had shown her that teas and luncheons were an impossible way to live. So she mapped out a schedule for herself, learned to cook, and took a business course. Never adrift, she now became fully engaged with pursuit of her own dreams. But Eleanor Roosevelt, like the rest of us, did not get to choose all the influences that would shape her life. She also had domestic emergencies that required her attention and personal resources.

The next year, Franklin came down with infantile paralysis, and she found that period to be the most difficult of her life. She argued with her mother-in-law over Franklin's care, but more important to her own development, she was forced to reconsider her role as the primary parent and provide a normal existence for her young boys. "I would have to become more of an all-round person than I had ever been before."[8]

During midlife, she found the courage to reclaim herself. At forty-nine years old she had faced her situation and arrived at the assessment that her early married life had been directed by her mother-in-law's values; her mothering years had been shaped to accommodate her husband and children's lives; and only now was she free to set her own course. When she had sent her last child off to school, she wanted to use her mind and abilities to achieve her own aims. "On the whole, I think I lived those years very impersonally. It was almost as though I had erected someone outside myself who was the President's wife. I was lost somewhere deep down inside myself."[9]

When Franklin Roosevelt died in 1945, Eleanor left the White House. She identified with all the other widows who faced a future alone, without a husband or children at home. For Eleanor, Franklin's death also meant that there was no one, except herself, to be the center of her life.

And in later years, looking back, she saw that, for much of her early life, she had been driven by the need to gain and keep the approval of others. Their love had been her aim. She had been timid and afraid. She had not considered any needs of her own, other than to be loved, and Eleanor did whatever was necessary to bring her closer to that goal. Then, in middle age, she found that "I had the courage to develop interests of my own. . . . And, having learned to stare down fear, I long ago reached the point where there is no living person whom I fear, and few challenges that I am not willing to face."[10]

To be sure, Eleanor Roosevelt is in the history books, having lived one of the more admirable lives of this century, but her story, despite the White House and the glamour, echoes working-class Shirley Valentine, who was pleased to finally be able to say, "She's there in the time she's livin' in." These women were engaged—first by their families, and then by a wider world. In midlife, they found courage to become involved in life in new ways. They were rewarded by gains in confidence.

Throughout the years, we get glimpses of who we are—vague at first, when we are young and eager to please, stronger with age and experience.

At midlife, most of us have an idea of who we are and who we are not, and this awareness allows us to move closer to an authentic self.

GENTLE TURNS IN THE ROAD

In high school, my driver's education teacher taught me to accelerate in turns. That advice seems to work best when the turns are gradual. The beginning of Melissa's awakening was conspicuously gentle and innocent. She said:

I went to graduate school and got a degree in social work and took a class in psychodynamic theory. [The professor] talked about learning disabilities as a disability that people couldn't see, yet it altered their view of the world because they processed information in a different way from the rest of the world. It was really the first time that I thought about myself—I have a hearing impairment. I began to think about how the hearing impairment impacted on my personality and my development.

A passing lecture, but one by a person she trusted and admired. She was, for unknown reasons, ready to think about her lifelong hearing impairment in a different way than ever before. This class encouraged her to get into therapy and address the influence of her hearing loss; it guided her later work with deaf people and shaped the years to follow. Choices are made one at a time. It is later, looking backward, that we are able to see the pattern.

For Kate, the turning point came when she was offered a promotion at work. She quit. The promotion meant that Kate had nothing left to prove; she had learned that she could earn a good living. As a lesbian it was important to her that she made it in a straight, intellectual environment; they accepted her, so "it seems like a very natural ending. . . . Others think getting a promotion and leaving might not seem like a natural ending, but it was reaching it that mattered, whatever happened." She got tired of looking for acceptance from others. Now she was going to get closer to an acceptance of herself. She had not wanted to leave her job as a failure, and now, with the promotion, she could leave as a success. Kate had already begun to look into other opportunities. She had a good support network and knew her next direction. Melissa's change was gradual, and Kate had laid the groundwork for her seemingly abrupt decision to quit her job. Those factors made their turning points gentle. Nevertheless, at the beginning, we cannot know the outcome.

We are motivated to change course by many forces, both internal and external. In Melissa there was curiosity. Kate was encouraged to leave her job because of unhappiness and discomfort. Both found the encounters inviting and took advantage of a new opportunity. We change when we are able. On the outside, we have, just as Eleanor Roosevelt did, mothers-in-law, husbands, careers, growing children, successes and failures, illnesses, and chance encounters that open doors. At midlife, we often summon up the courage to walk through those doors. Not all doors open gently, however.

HAIRPIN TURNS

Other turning points rudely shock us. Just as Eleanor Roosevelt could never have anticipated her husband's polio and the accommodations she would have to make to provide normal physical activities for their children, Bobbi could never have predicted that her son would become addicted to drugs. Bobbi and Ed had the perfect, high school–sweetheart marriage. Their plans had gone smoothly since they were eighteen. They went to the same university, Ed went to law school while Bobbi taught math, he built a prosperous law practice while she stayed home for a while, and when the kids were in school, Bobbi opened a shop. Their first son, Josh, was bright and musical. He was fifteen when the cops brought him home for selling crack. Bobbi had been blissfully unaware that Josh was a serious drug addict. All at once, her world collapsed; she had a different marriage and family, she had a diminished view of herself, and she had very real and serious adjustments to make. Ed was also stunned, but reacted by withdrawing into work; it took him years to accept the problem. Josh's illness depleted their financial and emotional resources and left their younger daughter furious at being pushed into family obscurity. Bobbi blamed herself for the family's problems, and Ed was willing to let her take on the emotional burdens while he concentrated on solutions to the financial responsibilities. After the shock wore off, Bobbi looked at the seriousness of the problem and took charge. She drew on strength she never knew she had, humor, good friends, and stubborn refusal to be defeated. She had never wanted the sickness, family problems, and financial worries, but since she could not change the situation, she changed her attitude. She mourned the loss of the perfect family and stuck with unpleasant reality. As she made decisions, even mistakes, she felt better and more confident that she could have some control over the situation rather than blindly reacting to her son's problems. She learned that she was a "survivor." Bobbi met the challenges and believes that she is all the better for it—confident, competent, and tested. Bobbi received no gentle invitation to grow or change. She was tossed into the nightmare and learned as she went along.

Strangely, a common thread links the turning points of each woman that I interviewed and the many women that I have treated in therapy over the years. In each encounter, some aspect of the problem resonated with a profound question inside the woman, engaged her, and pulled her to respond. That was the real cause of her change. These same events could have been presented to other women and been ignored. Every day, women go through experiences and remain untouched by them, but to be transforming, these encounters must hold on to us. For hearing-impaired Melissa, it was a need to come to terms with "being different." Bobbi, whose life had gone so smoothly, needed to know that she had the strength to rise to a challenge. Kate needed to know that she could succeed in the straight world before giving up an old wish to be accepted. These were unresolved personal concerns that were engaged by the event, figured in the work, led to more freedom, and offered the possibility of healing. Questions were answered; restraints were lifted: this is creative living.

Every creative encounter is a new event, and we start at the beginning. We connect to "the reality of experience," which is intensely personal.[11] To help foster our creative responses, we can try to be flexible, get rid of ready-made reactions, and remain open to our experience. Ready-made reactions, sameness, and apathy are protections designed to lessen the pain. But these responses also reduce the possibility for new and pleasant sensations. Sameness shelters us against both excitement and despair. When we can go beyond the self-protection and take the risk of exposing ourselves, we have the opportunity to move closer to our own psychological completeness, overcoming gaps and deficiencies that remain from our past experiences and development.

UPSETTING A BALANCE

For women who were not adventurous, turning points, at the very least, changed the light from "stop" to "go." In a comfortable niche at work and at home, Irene chafed but could not move. She was thirty-eight and conventional. She liked her old friends, her old dog, and her old job, all in the city in Wisconsin where she grew up. She took care of the books for a theater company, near the excitement but not in it. Since her divorce at thirty-three, she clung more closely than ever to stability. Then, in the year she turned thirty-nine, her closest friend was transferred to another state, her dog died, and she admitted that her job bored her. But life was familiar and she could not let any of it go. When the theater company folded, she was out of work overnight. Her first reaction was panic, and she interviewed for five local bookkeeping jobs within the week and got an offer. The job possibility reassured her that she could regain security. Then, calmer, Irene took many deep breaths and called her best friend. They talked. She began to see possibilities rather than losses. She had saved money, had skills, and realized that jobs were available. Her friend convinced her to come to Atlanta for a long visit, and when Irene returned, she was ready to examine new possibilities in different areas of her life. Her unemployment shoved her off her comfortable path, but it was her attitude that revealed the silver lining in the minidisaster.

When change is unwelcome, we cannot embrace it easily. Unwanted surprises expose us as unprepared, so reactions are initially fearful, and we try to reestablish the old ways. But even unwelcome events, because they upset the status quo, give us a chance to try new attitudes or behaviors. When the change is more internally motivated, or we are prepared, even unconsciously, we are emotionally more receptive to the work necessary to make the transition; some of the work has probably already been done.

TAKEN FROM US OR GIVEN UP

When Maria learned that her husband was having an affair and wanted a divorce, she threw up all day. When Christy decided to leave her husband, she cried all month. Both women's marriages ended, both grieved, and both went through feelings of fear, failure, and doubt. But the meaning of the separations were very different; one major distinction is that Maria's marriage ended by a decision that she did not make, whereas Christy exercised choice and gave up her marriage. Christy believed that she had power to take positive action in her life and leave a bad situation, but Maria said, "I felt so rejected and out of control." The decision was taken out of Maria's hands. There were similar outcomes to the marriages, maybe similar advantages and regrets, but very different paths, leaving each woman with a totally different sense of control. The turning points appeared in different guises. Some felt like gifts, others like toothaches, but these two women stayed through the process in order to refocus their lives.

RHYTHM OF CHANGE

Each of us has her own way to negotiate change. Some of us sit in an emotional swamp unconsciously working at change, and then the ideas and directions pop out of the muck; others of us ruminate and rehearse any proposed changes; some dwell on the fears; and some stay focused on the goals. We *all* get frustrated by our slowness in changing and imagine that everyone else cruises along at a fast pace. The empathy and compassion that we, as women, have traditionally had for others would be well spent on ourselves. Combined with knowledge of ourselves, compassion rather than harsh criticism helps us to understand our experiences, feel the emotions, and sit with our responses in a nonjudgmental way long enough to make clear decisions. It is easier to accept our lives when we have created them. We have increased difficulty when we feel that we are simply reacting to roles and events forced on us.

Many women are more comfortable old than young because youth had forced them into roles that were not altogether suitable for them. Perhaps the dutiful daughter, the stay-at-home mom, or the ambitious career woman was not a well-fitting identity. As we age, we are freed to adjust our roles to make them more suitable. Instead of one-size-fits-all, we can move to a designer life. My older cousin recently surprised me with the observation

"You were never conventional; you were just raised in a conventional home." I wish I had understood that thirty years ago. I would have been saved the lurking sense of being dropped into a play having memorized the wrong script.

LEARNING TO APPRECIATE SOLITUDE

Even with good support in place, crossroads remain a place where some decisions are made alone. Not every aspect of life can be shared with someone else or understood by another person. There are emotions and events that we experience alone, married or single, with children or without. Because of our emphasis on connections, being alone evokes fear. Women ask all the time, "Is there anything worse than being alone?" Yes, being estranged from ourselves is worse, because then we are truly alone. No number of people in the world can provide connection or comfort if we have lost ourselves. Creativity needs solitude. There are times when the questions and answers have to come from us and no one else. Turning points can be creative; they can also be frightening, in part because change makes us feel alone. Friends, family, loved ones, and professionals all can help, but there are still moments of solitude. As the women in these narratives moved through the process and became refocussed, they experienced solitude as a joy rather than a fear. Once they knew and trusted themselves, they enjoyed their own company. When they had confidence, they relished their own counsel. Solitude did not replace other people and the stimulation from outside, but solitude became a place to refresh themselves.

No one is able to tell us who we are better than we can—if we listen. Holly reflected on one turning point in her life and said, "It made me think about what did I really want, and I hadn't thought for a long time about what I really wanted. . . . I got into this path, working very hard and not thinking very hard about what I was doing—not making choices about it— about what I really want to do. . . . At some point . . . I began to think about what do I want to do and how do I want to live my life and what's important to me."

When we know who we are, when we love what we do, we may be alone, but being ourselves provides a sense of comfort and security. Authenticity cannot be a protection against sadness because it allows and includes all feelings that are real.

Change seems to follow a process that has three phases: first, the shake-up of the inner self occurs, as emerging potentials move into private thoughts and dreams; second, the newfound qualities are displayed to trusted friends or mentors; and third, the new endowments, now settled and possessed of direction, are shown to the world at large.[12]

Other people can help us—even kind voices from long ago bring encouragement—and in everyday life, we need supportive environments in which we give and receive hope and reassurance. Support keeps anxiety down and confidence up, although the choices ultimately are up to each one of us alone. Even in situations that we have not asked for and may not want, we have choices. After all else is gone, we are still left with "the last of human freedoms—the ability to choose one's attitude in a given set of circumstances."[13]

NOTES

Quote in chapter title is from the movie *The Rocky Horror Picture Show*.

1. Margery Williams, (1985), *The velveteen rabbit or how toys become real* (New York: Doubleday), p. 17.

2. Eleanor Roosevelt, (1958), *The autobiography of Eleanor Roosevelt* (New York: Harper & Brothers), pp. 61, 62.

3. Ibid., p. 62.

4. Ibid., p. 66.

5. Ibid., p. 90.

6. Ibid., p. 97.

7. Ibid., p. 103.

8. Ibid., pp. 117, 121.

9. Ibid., pp. 279, 280.

10. Ibid., p. 412.

11. Rollo May, (1975), *The courage to create* (New York: Norton), p. 20.

12. David Gutmann, (1987), *Reclaimed powers* (New York: Basic Books), p. 134.

13. Viktor Frankl, (1963), *Man's search for meaning* (New York: Washington Square Press), p. xiii.

❖ 13 ❖

"I HAVE A BRAIN AND A UTERUS AND I USE BOTH"
Women and Work

"We have not talked about the last book, the new one, the one which has brought us and the critics to sit at your feet. But at least I begin to understand what has gone into its making. So perhaps I begin to understand what you mean about 'women's work' too. At least I think *I do . . ." He paused and rubbed his forehead with one hand while he glanced back through his notes. "They have to write from the whole of themselves, so the feminine genius is the genius of self-creation. The outer world will never be as crucial for its flowering as the inner world, am I right?"*
  —May Sarton, *Mrs. Stevens Hears the Mermaids Singing*

Don't learn the tricks of the trade, learn the trade.
  —Anonymous

No longer diverted by other emotions, I work the way a cow grazes.
  —Kathe Kollwitz

Money speaks, but it speaks in a male voice.
  —Andrea Dworkin

To my surprise, when I found women who changed in their middle years, this growth was most often externally reflected in their work. Freud defined mental health as the ability "to love and to work." Many women agree with him.

Most of us are working now. In 1995, almost 59 percent of all American women over the age of 16 were in the civilian labor force, and the number is expected to rise to 60.6 percent by the year 2000 and 61.7 percent by 2005.[1] White women will provide the greatest number of additional working individuals.[2] In 1995, 77 percent of women between the ages of 35 and 44, and more than 74 percent of women between 45 and 54 years old, were in the labor force, and each of these percentages are projected to rise higher than 78 percent by 2000.[3] Married women (61 percent) are almost as likely as single women (66.8 percent) to be employed.[4] More than 70 percent of women with children under 18 years old and almost 61 percent of all mothers with children under the age of 6 worked for pay in 1995.[5] In 1960, married women with children made up 18.6 percent of the labor force, but in 1995, the percentage was up to 63.5.[6] These numbers mean a lot of legs are squeezing into panty hose each day. The news remains mixed. Many women work in the house, some trying to balance multiple responsibilities. They account for two-thirds of the 1.5 million people who work entirely in a home office.[7]

In 1992, women owned 33 percent of U.S. companies, but these businesses generated only 11 percent of the receipts.[8] A 1997 survey of corporate boards of Fortune 500 companies found that only 1 in 10.6 of their board members was female, but that is an increase of 18 percent of the seats since 1994.[9] In spite of inroads into traditionally male occupations, most jobs tend to be gender segregated, and by 1998, women still only made 76 cents for every dollar earned by men, up from 72 cents in 1990 and 63 percent in 1979.[10] In every occupation, women earned less than their male counterparts, ranging from 62 percent for production workers to 96 percent for registered nurses. Education helped, and women with at least a college degree came closest in earnings to their male counterparts, earning 77 percent of men's income, but women between the ages of 45 and 54 earned only two-thirds of men's income.[11] To be optimistic, earnings for women have increased faster than inflation, so we are moving forward.

Work has always been acknowledged as a significant part of a man's life. Psychologist Irene Stiver attempted to distinguish whether women's problems at work are different from men's problems and wrote:

What is immediately apparent is that for men, work has been a means of enhancing their experience of themselves as men, supporting their identities as men, and work has always been an important source of self-esteem. The successful man is perceived as more masculine than the man who is less successful. Many women, on the other hand, experience considerable conflict between their sense of self at work and their sense of self in their personal lives. Typically for women, work has not been a source of self-esteem.[12]

The women interviewed here felt differently. Although all women were acutely aware of the dizzying balance they had maintained for years, work was deeply meaningful to them. Particularly at midlife, women turn their increasing capacities for creativity and assertiveness into their work. The timing is good. In a study that sought to distinguish the productive years of life, seven hundred men and women were surveyed and researchers found that the twenties showed little productive work, the thirties improved, especially in art and literature, but the most productive decade was the period from 40 to 49, and for scholars, production continued into old age.[13]

Not all the women I interviewed were presently working full-time, and several were in work transitions. Work is important for many reasons, including self-esteem, but its primary value is that work provides money, and for us all, money is freedom. One woman remembered conversations from twenty-five years ago: "I'd say, 'Don't quit your job; money is important,' and my friends would say, 'It's a capitalistic trap to value money.'" Is it possible to make creative change with no resources? I am afraid it would be unbearably difficult. The women here were mostly college graduates and well-educated professionals, so they already had some value in the work-force. I was told the following story by one of them.

When I was a caseworker one year, between college and graduate school, I remember meeting an old woman who lived in a transient hotel. But in any case, she was a lovely woman, and her little room was full of trophies. She had been a nationally ranked golfer in the twenties, and she obviously came from a sort of Newport, high WASP family, and as I spoke to her, it transpired that she had been very well-to-do. She had gone into the hospital when she was about sixty and left her son with power of attorney. And he was a wastrel. And by the time she came out, everything was gone. For some reason, that anonymous woman's story so frightened me about my own money that I've always worked and I've always had private money. And I just think that freedom of choice for women is really rooted in having your own money. Also, of course, the determination that it is your own money. But I don't know what you do if you don't have money or an occupation. I don't mean money in the bank so much as the capacity.

JUGGLING MULTIPLE COMMITMENTS

For most of the women, career paths were not straight. For all the women, there was an endless juggling act of multiple responsibilities. All women grapple with the issue of how to balance family and work. Because relationships are so important to women, time away from children seems to take more of a toll on women than men. To hold on to both, we figure out a delicate stability between home and work. If anything upsets this equilibrium, such as a change in plans, new hours at work, or unexpected needs at home, we are thrown into terrible anxiety and feel that we have lost control of the situation. The conflicts are not only with the responsibilities for mothering. Women worry that their work will threaten their husbands. Women fear that competence leads to loneliness. It has been wryly noted that a successful man gets cared for, and a successful woman is considered to be someone who can take care of herself.[14]

When women work, they rarely give up other roles. Several studies have shown that women who chose occupational positions more like their fathers than their mothers did not relinquish domestic roles. Therefore, many women have combined the roles of their own mothers and fathers. This makes life complicated, but provides continuity of family values in terms of those roles. Women with careers describe their relationships with their own fathers to have increased tension and criticism but also increased understanding and support.[15]

Work gets easier in the middle years because we can attend to it with fewer interruptions for car pools and visits to pediatricians. The period when children are getting older coincides with our own comfort in feeling more aggressive and an increased sense of ourselves as capable adults. New ventures are possible at work that might be too chancy to try in other areas of life. Therefore, in the middle years, work can be part of completing old dreams or creating new ones. The artist Kathe Kollwitz wrote at age forty-three, "I am gradually approaching the period in my life when work comes first. When both the boys went away for Easter, I hardly did anything but work. Worked, slept, ate and went for short walks. But above all I worked."[16]

WORK REFLECTS GROWTH

We see that no decisions are pure; none is all healthy or all pathological. We enter our chosen fields for complex reasons, most of which are probably unknown to us at the time. Work can be entered for the wrong reasons and, once examined, still have enough healthy qualities in it to satisfy us for large portions of our lives; if not, we gather our courage and change.

Jenna's father refused to send her to college, and she had no idea of how to get there on her own. She accepted his view that she had limited capabilities and followed his instructions to get a secure but unchallenging job. At the other extreme in terms of parental advice, Lila's parents instilled in her the need to do something "important," preferably medicine, but law would have been acceptable. She went into medicine. Her sister studied law. Both Jenna and Lila resigned from their jobs. Jenna changed her work completely and painfully, but now works in sales with enthusiasm and initiative. She could afford to start over because she had not climbed very high. Lila does not know what to do. She had more invested and no alternative direction. Lila worried, "I would think to myself, really, who will I be without this job? What I've basically figured out is that I'm exactly the same person." The women I spoke with were all in different places in the process. Some women were able to stay in the same general field and expand, shift, or meander. Psychologists added consultation to their work, women in business moved into administration or policy making, and a few women got into research. These women have new challenges with the same basic identity. In a study of married, professional nurses in their early to late forties, all of whom valued personal growth, they began to see new possibilities, whether or not they would move into them. The career in nursing was, by midlife, part of their definition of themselves. They felt that they could grow within the general profession because they saw new opportunities.[17] Sometimes we have to begin new dreams in adulthood. But new dreams are not always new careers. Sometimes "new" is doing similar activities with a newfound understanding or motivation, or for pay instead of for free—wanting and choosing instead of going along for the ride.

Contrast these women with Melanie, now fifty. She was an artist, gave it up entirely for business, and has now returned to painting. Before she left her job, Melanie took off one month and went to Greece to reclaim herself as an artist. For the first weeks, she painted the house she lived in, rather than canvas, and then her art returned. The change is taking time. She had two distinct, nonoverlapping careers, both meaningful. She had regrets about leaving art, but there was no money in it. When she looked back and compared herself to a colleague who stayed in art, she found Helen to be "beaten down, bitter, struggling to survive as an artist; she has nothing. . . . I used to think it meant that she was smarter than me because she chose what she wanted to do and stuck with it, but then, when I saw the results of sticking with a losing situation, it didn't look so good. . . . It means a compromise or two along the way. . . . She is not an artist who has her heart in it anymore." Resuming work after a lapse meant that all Melanie had learned from other activities could be brought to use. She exemplifies the idea that we can have a network of ambitions that allows long-term goals, some of which may never be finished. We need to aspire high but work realistically.[18] There is no existing theory that allows a commitment to one or two major fields and the management of parallel and sometimes inter-related investments of time and love, and yet that is exactly the way most of us live our adult lives as women. Standard beliefs about work do not reflect the reality of women's lives; men's work lives are better understood. Unfortunately, this often causes us to feel that we have done something wrong rather than simply honor being different and feel confident that we are ahead of theory, not behind.

In the different paths taken by these women, we see again that we cannot live out other people's expectations of us, high or low. Maybe Lila still would not have stayed in medicine if it had been her choice, but perhaps she would have felt some ownership in becoming a doctor. When she failed to make the work her own, she got stuck. Lila never grew within her career, so options narrowed. Finally, she saw the only choices as to stay or to leave. In a study of midlife women who changed jobs, Rosalie Ackerman found four categories of attitudes and behaviors: Creators, who wanted change and made plans; Maintainers, who wanted change but made no plans; Con-ventionalists, who had not wanted change but made plans anyway; and Re-actors, who had not wanted change and made no plans. Not surprisingly, the Maintainers were the largest group. Most of us think about change but do not take much action. In work as well as in other areas of life, we adjust to change more easily when we have choices available. We are also helped by creative coping, which includes personal, psychological, and social re-sources to ease the strain of transitions. Self-esteem is important, and moderate optimism allows flexibility and keeps rigid responses to a minimum. The key to creative coping was the ability to generalize old learning to new situations in novel, flexible ways.[19]

Holly, forty-four, was touted to me as a total professional; she has a marvelous academic record and has had a series of excellent jobs culminating this year in a business partnership. Both men and women like to hire her, and subordinates adore her because she listens to them. To explain her history with regard to work, she needed to go back fifteen years. "That was a real turning point in my life, looking back." She lost a pregnancy and threw herself into work, "not thinking very hard about what I was doing—not making choices about it. I did what kind of came along to do." She was offered interesting, challenging positions, so she went along. "I really didn't have a plan. I didn't think about what is important to me. . . . I wasn't very ready to take too many risks. . . . My confidence in my ability was not that strong—I think it was a real competence issue." It was not until her forties, when she reconnected to beliefs from years earlier that had been swept aside by her busyness, that she gained clarity on "what kind of work environment I wanted to be in, realizing I wasn't going to have kids." The reconnection to old beliefs was strengthened when her husband started his own business. "I also thought, If he can do what he wants to do and take these risks, then I should do that too." Her career, which on the outside looks so clear and determined, in her view was a series of invitations until she reclaimed old beliefs. Then she could act on them.

SUCCESS

Concerning the relationship that women have with their work, the midlife refocus is directed to make work life-enhancing and nourishing. Leslie just stepped out into the air with faith that a good idea for a store could work. She had no specific training and no money—just a dream.

Leslie said:

I realized I love people. I love being around people. My fear was holding me back. . . . It just sounded scary, paying rent. . . . I felt, we're gonna go for it. I read every single book I could find written only by women on how to start a business, and I started my files. Step by step, the store began with one file folder on my desk, and it just kept growing, and I became more and more excited. . . . By March we started collecting inventory in our house. It was filled with inventory. We didn't have a store. Every room was filled with boxes except the bathroom.

Now, three years later, the store gives Leslie energy. "I mean, there are days that are very long and tiring, but it's all going in the direction that I want it to go. . . . I feel incredibly creative and the juices are always flowing;

there's always something exciting to do, you know, to make the store more appealing and comfortable for people."

Leslie and Holly are wonderful examples of the expansiveness possible when the production, such as one's work, is creative. As a result of their activity, Leslie and Holly have furthered their emotional development. When we try new behaviors and are successful, we begin to consolidate new self-images that are close to cherished ideals of ourselves.[20] Suitable work can help us grow in the direction of our fondest hopes; that is creativity's appeal. We become more like the women we want to be. All the women I have written about grew and gained access to aspects of themselves that were previously unavailable. In addition to enjoying new aspects of themselves, Leslie, Holly, and the others have work that involves communication and connection with people who want their products, whether the creations are art, social programs, business services, or information. Work enriches their lives, and other women report the same thing. Whether married, single, widowed, or divorced, work increases feelings of competence. Furthermore, older, intellectually gifted women who were single, divorced, or widowed for more than twelve years came out higher on scores of general happiness than married women because they had met the challenge of making their own lives.[21]

Our generations received consistent advice about work. First, the advice was "Be a teacher" or "Learn to type," which implied that our work would always be secondary to a husband's, and we ought to have something to fall back on, but we should not take our careers too seriously. I have taught for years and I know how to type; these suggestions disturb me because of the implied attitude, not the skills involved. Second, we were told to "fit in," or "Don't make waves." Again, there is nothing wrong with fitting in or learning to cooperate, but too often, those suggestions have been based on the belief that women's ways are second-best and need to be given up if we are to succeed. Lawyer Florynce Kennedy is quoted as saying, "There are very few jobs that actually require a penis or vagina,"[22] but to succeed in male domains, we are told, we must become more masculine, which means become more task oriented, think more analytically, hide emotion, and appear to have fewer personal reactions. Strong emotional tone, often quite comfortable for women, is perceived as demanding or hysterical by others, usually men. Communication then becomes difficult because men become anxious or reactive. It is still a male workplace, and emotions shown at the office are frowned upon. Often women's attempts to form relationships are mislabeled as expressions of dependency, whereas men are admired for "team building." Men are applauded when they show ambition; when women work toward their own advancement, they feel selfish and are often perceived that way by others. It is no wonder that women begin to believe that their styles are incompatible with existing organizational life.

Women may also define success differently than men do. Maybe a young lawyer does not want to work one hundred hours a week. Maybe that is not success; maybe success is an integration of meaningful work and connections. The choices we make at work are similar to other decisions. Preferences depend on who we are, what we need and want, and where we are in our lives. These directions are not right or wrong, but they are acutely personal.

NOTES

Quote in chapter title is from Pat Schroeder, when asked how she could be both a member of Congress and a mother, as quoted in L. Clark (Ed.), (1977), *Women women women: Quips, quotes and commentary* (New York: Drake), p. 53.

1. U.S. Bureau of the Census, *Statistical Abstract of the United States: 1996* (116th ed.), Washington, D.C., 1996, p. 393.

2. Ibid., p. 393.

3. Ibid., p. 393.

4. Ibid., p. 399.

5. Ibid., p. 400.

6. Ibid., p. 389.

7. Cynthia Costello and Barbara Kivimae Krimgold, (Eds.), (1996), *The American woman: 1996–1997* (New York: Norton), p. 63.

8. U.S. Department of Commerce, Bureau of the Census. www.census.gov

9. Catalyst women.org

10. Usual weekly earnings summary, April 20, 1998. Labor force statistics from the current population survey. Bureau of Labor Statistics cpsinfo@bls.gov

11. Costello and Krimgold, (Eds.), *The American woman,* pp. 66–67.

12. Irene P. Stiver, (1991), Work inhibitions in women, in J. Jordan, A. Kaplan, J. Baker Miller, I. Stiver, and J. Surrey (Eds.), *Women's growth in connection: Writings from the Stone Center* (New York: Guilford Press), p. 224.

13. Wayne Dennis, (1968), Creative productivity between the ages of 20 and 80 years, in B. Neugarten (Ed.), *Middle age and aging* (Chicago: University of Chicago Press), pp. 106–14.

14. Stiver, Work inhibitions in women, p. 226.

15. C. Nydegger and L. Mitteness, (1991), Fathers and their adult sons and daughters, *Marriage and Family Review* 16:249–56.

16. Kathe Kollwitz, (1974), quoted in Mary Jane Moffat and Charlotte Painter (Eds.), (1974), *Revelations: Diaries of women* (New York: Random House), p. 199.

17. Virginia Olesen, (1990), Self-assessment and change in one's profession: Notes on the phenomenology of aging among mid-life women, *Journal of Women and Aging* 2(4):69–79.

18. Doris Wallace, (1985), Giftedness and the construction of a creative life, in F. D. Horowitz and M. O'Brien (Eds.), *The gifted and talented: Developmental perspectives* (Washington, DC: American Psychological Association), pp. 361–84.

19. Rosalie Ackerman, (1990), Career developments and transitions of middle-aged women, *Psychology of Women Quarterly* 14:513–30.

20. Milton Viederman, (1988), Personality change through life experience 111:

Two creative types of response to object loss, in D. Dietrich and P. Shabad (Eds.), *The problem of loss and mourning: Psychoanalytic perspectives* (New York: International Universities Press), pp. 187–212.

21. Pauline Sears and Ann Barbee, (1977), Career and life satisfaction among Terman's gifted women, in J. Stanley, W. George, and C. Solano (Eds.), *The gifted and creative: Fifty-year perspective* (Baltimore: Johns Hopkins University Press), pp. 28–65.

22. Florynce Kennedy, quoted in L. Clark (Ed.), *Women women women*, p. 51.

❖ 14 ❖

"LET THE BEAUTY YOU LOVE
BE WHAT YOU DO"
Achievements and Dreams

If you want your dreams to come true, don't sleep.
—Yiddish proverb

How many cares one loses when one decides not to be something, but to be someone.
—Coco Chanel, fashion designer

To me the sea is like a person—like a child that I've known a long time. It sounds crazy, I know, but when I swim in the sea, I talk to it. I never feel alone when I'm out there.
—Gertrude Ederle, first woman to swim the English channel

All the women I spoke with achieved a great deal; most notably, they had taken responsibility for the shape and direction of their lives. They faced and accepted necessary losses, and in doing so, they found space within themselves and in their lives. The fear of emptiness was tolerated until, in the clarity of that space, the women saw the directions in which to refocus their energy. As the process of relinquishing, reconnecting, and refocussing drew to a close, the women described a synchronicity in their feelings and actions. The internal woman who holds thoughts, feelings, and beliefs and the woman who acts blended better than ever before. The past flowed into and informed the present, but did not rule. The women had transformed the dreams and passions of childhood into viable adult lives. They experienced a sense of freedom different from any they had known. However, the way I saw these women was obviously from my own perspective. A line in a Margaret Atwood poem reads, "The moon seen from the moon is a very different thing."[1] I wondered what the women themselves considered to be their achievements thus far, how they lived today, and what constituted their dreams.

GENERATIVITY

When asked to consider their achievements, most of the women who had children mentioned their sons and daughters first, and said, for example, in honest fashion, "Raising my children. Not killing them." One woman replied, "I think my greatest achievement is that my children love each other and are close." Another said, "I like their values. They are do-gooders and they care about people. They are close to my mother. They are funny." Still another said, "Having raised the children was a solid achievement." The women with older children had the pleasure of seeing them become loving, responsible adults. Whatever else mothers achieve, the healthy development of our children contributes to our sense of accomplishment because motherhood is an intense personal investment. My friend Nancy used to wonder about her five children, "Do you think the only memories that they'll have of me is that I told them to clean their rooms?" We want to have passed along more than household hints.

The roots of mothering lie in our own early development, so when the children are launched with success, it is the realization of an early, long-held ideal—to be a good mother. As our children grow, we also have the opportunities to soothe old wounds and reconcile conflicts from our pasts. Our own childhoods cannot be erased or lived again, but healing occurs when we do not repeat old mistakes with our children. In these ways, we are enhanced by their growth. We can feel gratified by the results of our years of hard work. These are significant achievements and realizations of dreams.

Among those I interviewed, for women who had children as well as for women who did not, the ability to guide and nurture people gave each one a sense of lasting accomplishment. They were proud of their flair for mentoring others in their professional lives. One woman offered, "I think the thing I'm most proud about is that I really advanced people. I gave people breaks." Many others also developed people and programs: "What I did at the school [is one of my proudest achievements]. I somehow always maintained my personal integrity while I was there, which was not an easy thing to do. I had a lot of impact on a lot of people's lives, and I think that was important." These creative achievements, generative in the deepest sense of the word, nourished the midlife women as well as the people who benefited from their generosity. We live in the people we guide, the programs we develop, and the works of all kinds that we create, and we last beyond what we alone can reach in one lifetime.

Often relationships with family and friends were noted as achievements. One woman, when asked about her greatest accomplishments, said, "The fact that I've been married for nineteen years." Another remarked, "I'm pleased that I'm close to my mother and my best friends. I have very dear friendships. That gives me a tremendous sense of confidence." When so much in our culture is fleeting and disposable, enduring marriages, family ties, and relationships with friends are a source of self-respect. They prove to us that we can go long distances. Enduring relationships bring to mind words that had no meaning in the vocabulary of my youth—grace, dignity, respect, and integrity.

AUTHENTICITY

Some of the women's greatest achievements were not about others, but about themselves and their lives today. "I keep changing. . . . Some people are ossified, and you see it spiral into a kind of narrow life. I think that's very frightening, and I haven't done it." Another said, "I've gotten to this place psychologically. I do feel stronger and healthier. I can rise to an occasion." They were proud of their continuing psychological growth and ability to venture out, take risks, and change. "I have confidence. I'm not going to go through life afraid," said a number of women. They wanted to continue to pursue only activities that had meaning. "A lot of people spend time trying to 'prove' who they are. That's not the question anymore. I just am," said one woman. Those feelings were echoed by comments such as, "I'm living free." More poignantly, one interviewee said, "I was a donkey [and a work animal for everyone else]. . . . Now, I savor small moments like the light shining in the window for as long as I want." They cared that they had made a difference, but the women no longer needed to please everybody and had less need to conform to other people's expectations. They were less willing to bother with nonessentials and had a firm grasp on their priorities. They valued their abilities to "accept" and "let go." Less harm comes to us from losses than from having no attachments. They became more whole because all aspects of their personalities were free to be expressed—young and old, passive and aggressive, strong and weak, talented and inept. They took risks. The fullness kept the women feeling vital and alive.

At midlife, we integrate all aspects of our personality, including the dark or shadow sides of ourselves. We could not have done it earlier because we were struggling to develop identities, and that forced us to concentrate on certain personality attributes and neglect others. Perhaps we emphasized nurturing or pleasing others, important qualities as young lovers, wives, or mothers. The earlier years were shaped by choices we made as to the roles we would assume, such as mother, wife, or career woman. In the past, we repudiated certain qualities because we saw them as undesirable, as the enemy, or as punishment to our good selves. Self-interest, anger, and indifference to others are common qualities that women treat as deficits, jettison early, and reclaim in midlife. If we continue to repudiate aspects of ourselves, we become less flexible, and we calcify rather than expand. Fighting with ourselves takes inordinate amounts of energy that might be directed in more useful work. In the stages of mourning and reconnection, we addressed the imbalance and brought our neglected qualities into consciousness, integrated them into ourselves. Maturity allows us to accept these qualities rather than to keep them at a distance and see them only in others, because we come to believe that the qualities we cherish—strength, integrity, kindness, and love—will keep the balance tipped in favor of lives of which we can be proud. The other qualities will remain the smaller, spicy aspects of ourselves.

The women I have written about worked hard and well. They honestly faced their losses and let them go to the extent that was possible. They reconnected with *all* aspects of themselves. It is in being complete, not perfect, that the women felt good about themselves. They also recognized and accepted limitations—of themselves, those they love, and of the world in which we all live. Further, they came to know the value of limits as well as their futility. Creativity requires limits, because the creative act is a struggle to transcend whatever limits us. In creative living, we go beyond our preset boundaries and enlarge our confines. These women achieved an expansiveness in their middle years. Most important, in order to do this, they had the courage to take risks, to make honest efforts, fully cognizant of the limitations of adulthood. They took hold of their lives in a world that is neither fair nor controllable. With the acceptance of this knowledge, the days became their own creations.

Achievements were successes in mothering and mentoring, relationships, and creative programs and products. Achievements were feeling confident, strong, knowing themselves and pleasing themselves, acceptance of some limits and pushing against others. What was important was not appearance but authenticity.

DREAMS

The adult dream embraces images of our ambitions and aspirations, a vision of how we wish to be in the adult world. The dreams fill us with excitement and energy. In the work of reconnecting to ourselves, we identify dreams, and in refocussing the future, we act on dreams.

The idea of an adult dream was originally used by Levinson in his 1978 study of midlife men.[2] The dream contains images of our central life goal. Recently, when the dream was examined in midlife women, it was found that women who had not formed a dream or who had given up a dream were more vulnerable to anxiety. Self-esteem or a sense of identity is enhanced by a successful dream. The researchers also found that women's dreams were more multifaceted than those of men, including a combination of marriage and family, career, and personal goals. The primacy of relational elements declines in midlife, but the personal dream continues to include images of personal growth, fulfillment of personal desires, and idiosyncratic individual goals that cannot be easily categorized in societal roles.[3]

One of the pressures of midlife is the idea that this is the last opportunity to make dreams come true. We cannot continue to hold images of ourselves that we do not live. Midlife is a time when health, vitality, and self-confidence are high; we know that aging lies invariably ahead, so some of us become increasingly willing to venture. When I had just turned forty-six, my doctor found a tumor; it was removed and found to be benign. At first I was overwhelmed by the relief and gratitude that comes with a close call, but about three months later, I had another idea. I realized that although I had been let off, I had been touched by the threat of cancer, and I thought, "One day it will be true; maybe not for a long time, but one of these days." That certainly urged me to set out in a few new directions—not to wait for anyone or anything. The same questions of What do I want? and When will I go after it? are with us throughout life; perhaps they gain a measure of urgency now. The sadness and hopelessness some women experience in the middle years does not come from trying and failing, but from not trying.

Any anxiety about mortality that we feel in the middle years may slow creative actions, but conversely, mortality may inspire a courageous surge to affirm life. Creativity, in the broadest sense, takes on new depths and shades of feeling, and under good circumstances, our creations are experienced as life-giving and comforting.[4]

The dreams that gave birth to nourishing productions had a common root. All had deep personal meaning in the lives of the women who pursued them. The women called their dreams fulfilling, meaningful, fun, empowering, and energizing. The women I spoke with moved in different directions to get closer to their dreams. A few of the women had been divorced, and some of them remarried; most women made adjustments in their relationships to partners, children, and friends. Several returned to art or changed art forms, several changed work, a few began businesses based on specific talents and interests, a couple of women adopted or gave birth to a first child, and several shifted within their work to projects or environments that were more representative of them. These creations came out of dreams and required acts of faith that something better was possible. Other women stayed put, and once they understood their motives, needs, and options with respect to love or work, the decision to remain in place was genuine; their journeys were more about making choices and less about making changes. For all of us, once we have made the internal journey where feelings and ideas are understood, even home is a new place.

The women in these pages have accomplished what other women have done before them and what many others can do now. As adult women, we have become tired of being told that we are dysfunctional and need to be fixed. What started out as a celebration of women's differences has again turned to deficits, and bookstore shelves are filled with ideas for getting us into shape, physically and emotionally. All this fixing is to make us more appealing—but to whom? The women I interviewed said that they wanted to enjoy life more and have fun. Creative living requires us to retain humor and the capacity to play. The women liked themselves again; they were not weighed down by the responsibilities of their lives, but were able to choose activities that they enjoyed; they fully intended to fill their days with people and work that they loved.

Dreams contain pictures that show us the way. When we take steps in those directions, updated for adulthood, we feel good. At midlife, our sense of mortality can help move us along, and failure becomes lack of effort, not lack of success. There is no rush; we can take a step at a time, pausing to listen to our own voices, which will tell us when to rest, when to redirect our efforts, and when to dance forward.

TRANSFORMATION OF DREAMS

The importance of dreams does not waver, although not all dreams last forever, and many dreams continued to evolve and change shape or direction. There is a completeness and a beauty intrinsic to our work when we do what we love. It has nothing to do with the outcome; the beauty is in the engagement. Although we give up illusions at midlife because holding on to them stops us from living life, we still need dreams. As children and adolescents, most of us had dreams of our future selves and the lives we would lead. These childhood dreams got lost in the day-to-day work of adult lives. Some women, in adulthood, take the opportunity to reconnect to the meaning of their dreams, if not the exact dreams themselves. They create new, adult dreams to point them in new directions.

In shaping our dreams, we must reach inside to find what we want to do, who we want to be, and what we are emotionally committed to, because when dreams include goals that increase personal competence or require new learning, we usually enjoy our efforts or performances. When we pursue activities for their intrinsic interest, simply because we want to, we are likely to become and remain fascinated and absorbed by them. In adults, intrinsic motivation has been shown to contribute to active, productive engagement in work, play, and creative activities. Conversely, when dreams are based on seeking favorable judgments from others, we respond poorly and give up more easily, avoid challenges, experience anxiety, and have lowered self-esteem. Concentrating on the external rewards decreases emotional involvement and increases negative feelings.[5]

Dreams serve as guides because old dreams may speak to the heart of who we still remain. Even if becoming a rock star is out, tap dancing is in. Dreams do not have to turn into careers; dreams give us back aspects of ourselves that provide joy and satisfaction. As we mature, we constantly reshape our personal and unique dreams and fantasies, which can be seen unhealthily in neuroses, but which also can direct our most satisfying and creative work. Creativity, then, is a lifelong process, that may find novel expression in different phases of our lives. Adult creativity may depict child and adolescent wishes in a more satisfactory way.[6] Much that had been neglected can be reshaped and reclaimed.

An illustration of the transformation of dreams can be found in the story of Eugene Lang, who, as a wealthy sixty-two-year-old, began the I Have a Dream Program, which funds college for high schoolers. This major project sprung out of a talk he was giving to poor students when he made the spontaneous offer of payment for the college education for each teen who graduated from high school. In tracing this unplanned action backward, we see that these were ideals that started in Lang's childhood with concrete goals, then shifted to abstract principles in adolescence, and shifted back, at midlife, to a level of generality in which he believed his own life might make a difference.[7] Old fantasies may never be extinguished, but may persist and manifest in a variety of forms throughout the life cycle. The middle years provide maturity, confidence, and the ability to go back to the fantasies and realize them in new ways.

We may see a blending of interests or the motivation to heal a special wound. Years ago, I interviewed mothers whose children had died, and there were some startling similarities among the activities of certain adaptive women who had worked hard for five or six years to make their way through this terrible loss. The women's lives were reorganized, and the loss had become integrated into their total identities. Still, the women had developed some new creative activities that allowed them to continue to work through the loss in a manner that let them remember the child, but fitted the personality of the mother. One creative woman whose daughter had been theatrically talented developed puppet shows to produce for other children. Another woman, who had talents for organization, had lost an athletic son. She established a living memorial in the form of scholarships for other young athletes. A nurse who had underestimated the severity of her daughter's illness put together workshops for hospital workers where the employees were trained to recognize and assist grieving family members. As they worked through their losses, energy was freed to be redirected in creative ways that satisfied their personalities and talents and addressed the loss. The creative directions never made their losses disappear, but it helped the women to mend. In the process of tending to their dreams to complete their unfinished mothering, these women reshaped their lives and offered their creations to others.

Creativity is often the outcome of successful mourning. Sometimes creativity may be an attempt to complete the mourning work, to repair or reinstate the loss, as in the case of these mothers. Creative work heals; it does not impoverish the creator but nourishes her, and thus more creative work is possible. Ideas, creations, and choices that we seem to reach rapidly and easily in adulthood are commonly themes that we have worked on before or that may have been emerging slowly over the years. For example, my own first book was about loss in women's lives and their adaptation to trauma. Over the last fifteen years, that theme has evolved to creativity and optimal outcomes in life adjustment. The creative products of today have their roots in the issues we worked through years before, so today we can often move ahead with greater ease and certainty. Themes of our lives are worked and reworked with increasing maturity and progress.

Even the mediums with which we work may change during our adulthood. Isabelle began as a fine art photographer, moved to portraits to capture the substance of her subjects, and is writing because she wants to go further. In a similar vein, research has demonstrated that composers and poets emerge successfully in young adulthood, whereas sculptors rarely achieve greatness until later. It is thought that music and words, as mediums for creative work, are much more amenable to the passion of rapid creativity than is the stone needed for sculpture. With stone, the working relationship to the material itself is important and demands a process of working over the product. There is an ability to engage differently, to have a relationship with the product, to work and rework the product. We have more discipline in our middle years, which permits the necessary patience. The restraint produces an interplay between intuitive work and rational consideration of the creation.[8] We have a relationship—not dominance, but interplay—with whatever we produce.

The creations of adulthood have a philosophical tone that approaches more of a serene state. The essence of creations in mature adulthood is that the innovation is not simply the end product or nearly the end product, but is instead a point in the process, to be modified or elaborated upon. There is greater appreciation of the moment; there is greater appreciation of the process and less rushing toward the goal. This speaks to the changed attitude toward time that occurs in the middle years, with its increased appreciation of the present. When we were young, we often looked longingly to the future, waiting for "life to begin."

Virginia Woolf, at forty-nine, on completing *The Waves*, is quoted as saying, "What interests me in the last stage was the freedom and boldness with which my imagination picked up, used and tossed aside all the images, symbols which I had prepared. I am sure that this is the right way of using them—not in set pieces, as I had tried at first, coherently, but simply as images, never making them work out; only suggest."[9] This is a good description of the later steps in the process of creative change. There is a speed and excitement as the pieces fall into place, a sense of fun that may have been missing during the introspective mourning and reconnection. Each bit of freedom is to be enjoyed. We have earned it, and pleasure in an expanded life will keep us repeating the process of relinquishing, reconnecting, and refocusing, which is depicted in Figure 9.

Artists provide the world with creative works in art, music, science, and other fields. For the less artistic, there is something that we have called creative living, which requires a similar capacity to transform the sludge of our lives into something better. This assertion of our dreams and our commitment to them is essential in order to keep reality in our lives. A woman

Refocused

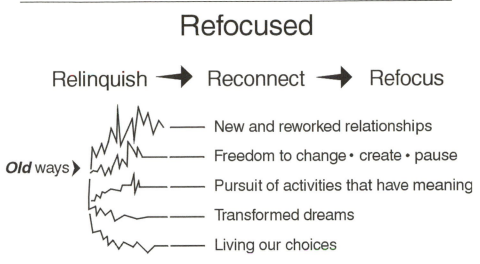

Relinquish ➜ Reconnect ➜ Refocus

New and reworked relationships

Freedom to change • create • pause

Old ways ❯ Pursuit of activities that have meaning

Transformed dreams

Living our choices

becomes fully human only by her choices and her commitment to them. We attain worth and dignity by the multitude of decisions we make each day.[10] We create ourselves by our thoughts and dreams and choices. We give form to our dreams when we are living creative lives. We are not simply engaged in knowing our world; we are engaged in a passionate reforming of our world by virtue of our interrelationship with it. Our reality is expanded. We further our emotional development and feel more complete as a result of creative activity. We grow; that is some of creativity's appeal.

The last word goes to Melanie: "I used to think that if I tried something and failed, I couldn't deal with the failure. I thought that I always had to be perfect. . . . I never competed in sports because I couldn't stand losing. If I didn't think I could win, I didn't go for it. That's how competitive I was. Tim pointed it out—I won't even play if I don't think I can win. Then I said, 'Wait a minute. I can live through it if I lose. I'm strong enough.' "

NOTES

Quote in chapter title is from A great wagon, in *The essential Rumi* (1995), translated by Coleman Barks (New York: Harper San Francisco), p. 36.

1. Margaret Atwood, (1978), Fortelling the future, in *Two-headed poems* (New York: Simon & Schuster), p. 12.

2. Daniel Levinson, (1978), *The seasons of a man's life* (New York: Alfred A. Knopf).

3. Charles Drebing, Hendrika Van de Kemp, Winston Gooden, and H. Newton Malony, (1995), The dream in midlife women: Its impact on mental health, *International Journal of Aging and Human Development* 40(1):73–87.

4. Elliot Jaques, (1981), The midlife crisis, in S. Greenspan and G. Pollack

(Eds.), *The course of life* 3:1–23 (Washington, DC: U.S. Department of Health and Human Services).

5. National Advisory Mental Health Council, (1995, October), Basic behavioral science research for mental health: A national investment, emotion and motivation, Rockville, MD, *American Psychologist* 50(10):843.

6. H. Peter Hildebrand, (1990), The other side of the wall: A psychoanalytic study of creativity in later life, in R. Nemiroff and C. Colarusso (Eds.), *New dimensions in adult development* (New York: Basic Books), p. 471.

7. Elizabeth Auchincloss and Robert Michels, (1989), The impact of middle age on ambitions and ideals, in J. Oldham and R. Liebert (Eds.), *The middle years: New psychoanalytic perspectives* (New Haven: Yale University Press), p. 50.

8. Jaques, The midlife crisis.

9. Virginia Woolf, (1974), in M. J. Moffat and C. Painter (Eds.), *Revelations: Diaries of women* (New York: Random House), pp. 193–94.

10. Rollo May, (1975), *The courage to create* (New York: Norton), p. 5.

❖ ❖ ❖

EPILOGUE

It has been more than six years since I conducted the first interview for this book. I have kept in touch with some of the women whose stories appear here. I have also heard snippets about the lives of others. When I heard news that was not the information I expected, my impulse was to rush back to the manuscript and edit out the story. I have not done that.

Melanie (pages 8–15), who quit work to return to art, has opened up her own business doing work very similar to the development work that she used to do, but now the business is her own and she plans to bring in her daughter as a partner. She also sent me an invitation to her art show. Nan (pages 25–26) did not marry after all. I don't know why. Isabelle (pages 34–37) continues to work full time teaching photography and writes as often as she can. Megan, first married at forty-three (pages 75–77), had her first child and is a stay-at-home mom after all these years of work. Con (page 114) happily moved to Europe for a job. Margaret (pages 160–162) came back into therapy briefly because her drinking threatened to get out of control. Claire's (pages 117, 147–148) business continues to thrive and is becoming quite well known. Laura's (pages 118–120) business folded with a loss of money and confidence, and although that year was one of her most difficult, she has moved into other satisfying, well-chosen opportunities. Bobbi (pages 176–177) has become a tougher woman than she used to be, in part because her son almost died before he gave up drugs. He is now clean and the family feels like they are all recovering. Karen (page 45) and Lila (page 184) both went back to part-time work in the same fields, work they disliked, but each has less responsibility and more freedom. And I have a contract to write another book.

So, was I wrong? Many women fell short of the goals that they described to me six years ago. But I don't think I am mistaken about the process. Each woman says that she is more alive, more in control of her world, and more engaged with life. Laura reminded me that success is not simply achieveng the goal, it is the attitude we take when we go after the dream.

❖ ❖ ❖

BIBLIOGRAPHY

Abzug, B., with M. Kelber. (1984). *Gender gap*. Boston: Houghton Mifflin.

Ackerman, R. (1990). Career developments and transitions of middle-aged women. *Psychology of Women Quarterly* 14:513–30.

Andreasen, N. (1987).Creativity and mental illness: Prevalence rates in writers and their first-degree relatives. *American Journal of Psychiatry* 144:1288–92.

Applegarth, A. (1986). Women and work. In T. Bernay and D. Cantor (Eds.), *The psychology of today's woman: New psychoanalytic visions*, pp. 211–30. New York: The Analytic Press.

Atwood, M. (1978). *Two-headed poems*. New York: Simon & Schuster.

Auchincloss, E., and R. Michels. (1989). The impact of middle age on ambitions and ideals. In J. Oldham and R. Liebert (Eds.), *The middle years: New psychoanalytic perspectives*, pp. 40–57. New Haven: Yale University Press.

Baker, S. J. (1992). Fighting for life. In J. K. Conway (Ed.), *Written by herself*, pp. 143–70. New York: Vintage Books.

Barnett, R. C., and G. K. Baruch. (1978). Women in the middle years: A critique of research and theory. *Psychology of Women Quarterly* 3(2):187–98.

Barron, F. (1963). Diffusion, integration, and enduring attention to the creative process. In R. W. White (Ed.), *The study of lives*, pp. 234–48. New York: Atherton Press.

Bateson, M. C. (1989). *Composing a life*. New York: Plume Press.

Baum, L. F. (1979). *The wizard of Oz*. New York: Ballantine Books. Original work published 1900.

Baumeister, R., and M. R. Leary. (1995). The need to belong: Desire for interpersonal attachments as a fundamental human motivation. *Psychological Bulletin* 117(3):497–529.

Begley, S. (1993, June 28). The puzzle of genius. *Newsweek*, pp. 46–51.

Black, S. M., and C. E. Hill. (1984). The psychological well-being of women in their middle years. *Psychology of Women Quarterly* 8:282–92.

Block, J. (1972). Generational continuity and discontinuity in the understanding of societal rejection. *Journal of Personality and Social Psychology* 22:333–45.

Brown, J. (1992). Lives of middle-aged women. In V. Kerns and J. K. Brown (Eds.), *In her prime: A new view of middle-aged women*, 4th ed., pp. 17–30. Urbana and Chicago: University of Illinois Press.

Bruch, C. B., and J. A. Morse. (1972, Winter). Initial study of creative (productive) women under the Bruch-Morse model. *Gifted Child Quarterly* 16:282–89.

Cameron, J. (1992). *The artist's way: A spiritual path to higher creativity*. New York: Tarcher/Perigee.

Campbell, J. (1964). *Myths to live by*. New York: Bantam.

Cangelosi, D., and C. E. Schaefer. (1992). Psychological needs underlying the creative process. *Psychological Reports* 71:321–22.

Cavafy, C. P. (1992). *C. P. Cavafy collected poems.* G. Savides (Ed.). Princeton: Princeton University Press.

Chafe, W. H. (1991). *The paradox of change: American women in the twentieth century.* New York: Oxford University Press.

Chasseguet-Smirgel, J. (1984). Thoughts on the concept of reparation and the hierarchy of creative acts. *International Review of Psychoanalysis* 11:399–409.

Chiriboga, D. A. (1981). The developmental psychology of middle age. In J. Howell (Ed.), *Modern perspectives in the psychiatry of middle age,* pp. 3–25. New York: Brunner\Mazel.

Chiriboga, D. A., and M. Thurnher. (1975). Concept of self. In M. Lowenthal, M. Thurnher, D. Chiriboga, and associates (Eds.), *Four stages of life: A comparative study of men and women facing transitions,* pp. 62–83. San Francisco: Jossey-Bass.

Chodorow, N. (1989). *Feminism and psychoanalytic theory.* New Haven: Yale University Press.

Chopin, K. (1972). *The awakening.* New York: Avon Books. Original work published 1899.

Clark, L. (Ed.). (1977). *Women women women: Quips, quotes, and commentary.* New York: Drake.

Cohler, B., and R. Galatzer-Levy. (1990). Self, meaning, and morale across the second half of life. In R. Nemiroff and C. Colarusso (Eds.), *New dimensions in adult development,* pp. 214–59. New York: Basic Books.

Cohler, B., and M. Lieberman. (1979). Personality change across the second half of life: Findings from a study of Irish, Italian and Polish-American men and women. In D. Gelfand and A. Kutznik (Eds.), *Ethnicity and aging,* pp. 227–45. New York: Springer.

Cohler, B., and F. Stott. (1988). Separation, interdependence, and social relations across the second half of life. In J. Bloom-Feshbach, S. Bloom-Feshbach, and associates (Eds.), *The psychology of separation and loss: Perspectives on development, life transitions, and clinical practice,* pp. 165–204. San Francisco: Jossey-Bass.

Coles, R. (1970). *Erik Erikson: The growth of his work.* Boston: Little, Brown.

Conway, J. K. (Ed.). (1992). *Written by herself.* New York: Vintage Books.

Costello, C., and B. K. Krimgold (Eds.). (1996). *The American woman 1996–1997: Where we stand.* New York: Norton.

Dennis, W. (1968). Creative productivity between the ages of 20 and 80 years. In B. Neugarten (Ed.), *Middle age and aging,* pp. 106–14. Chicago: University of Chicago Press. Original work published 1966.

Dixon, J., M. Hickey, and J. Dixon. (1992). A causal model of the way emotions intervene between creative intelligence and conventional skills. *New Ideas in Psychology* 10(2):233–51.

Drebing, C., H. Van de Kemp, W. Gooden, and H. Malony. (1995). The dream in midlife women: Its impact on mental health. *International Journal of Aging and Human Development* 40(1):73–87.

Edelstein, L. (1984). *Maternal bereavement.* New York: Praeger.

Edelstein, L. (1995). Creative change as a result of midlife mourning. Paper presented at the 103rd Annual Convention of the American Psychological Association, New York, NY.

Edelstein, L. (1997). Revisiting Erikson's views on generativity. Paper presented at the 104th Annual Meeting of the American Psychological Association, Chicago, IL.

Erikson, E. (1950). *Childhood and society*. New York: Norton.

Erikson, E. (1959). Identity and the life cycle. *Psychological Issues*, 1(1).

Evans, R. (1967). *Dialogue with Erik Erikson*. New York: Harper & Row.

Fiske, M. (1982). Challenge and defeat: Stability and change in adulthood. In L. Goldberger and S. Breznitz (Eds.), *Handbook of stress: Theoretical and clinical aspects*, pp. 529–43. New York: Free Press.

Frankl, V. (1963). *Man's search for meaning*. New York: Washington Square Press.

French, M. (1977). *The women's room*. New York: Summit.

Freud, S. (1957a). Female sexuality. In *Standard edition* 21:223–46. London: Hogarth Press. Original work published 1931.

Freud, S. (1957b). Mourning and melancholia. In *Standard edition* 14:243–58. London: Hogarth Press. Original work published 1917.

Friedan, B. (1983). *The feminine mystique*. New York: Dell. Original work published 1963.

Gabbard, G. O. (1993). On hate in love relationships: The narcissism of minor differences revisited. *Psychoanalytic Quarterly* 62:229–38.

Gilligan, C. (1982). *In a different voice*. Cambridge, MA: Harvard University Press.

Gilovich, T., and V. H. Medvec. (1995). The experience of regret: What, when and why. *Psychological Review* 102(2):379–95.

Gould, R. (1978). *Transformation: Growth and change in adult life*. New York: Simon & Schuster.

Greenacre, P. (1957). The childhood of the artist. In *Psychoanalytic study of the child* 12:47–72. New York: International Universities Press.

Gutmann, D. (1987). *Reclaimed powers*. New York: Basic Books.

Harris, R., A. Ellicott, and D. Holmes. (1986). The timing of psychosocial transitions and changes in women's lives: An examination of women aged 45 to 60. *Journal of Personality and Social Psychology* 51(2):409–16.

Hazan, C., and P. R. Shaver. (1994). Attachment as an organizational framework for research on close relationships. *Psychological Inquiry* 5:1–22.

Heilbrun, C. (1991, Summer). Naming a new rite of passage. *Smith Alumnae Quarterly*, pp. 26–28.

Helson, R., V. Mitchell, and G. Moane. (1984). Personality and patterns of adherence and nonadherence to the social clock. *Journal of Personality and Social Psychology* 46:1079–96.

Helson, R., and G. Moane. (1987). Personality change in women from college to midlife. *Journal of Personality and Social Psychology* 53(1):176–86.

Helson, R., and P. Wink. (1992). Personality change in women from the early 40s to the early 50s. *Psychology and Aging* 7(1):46–55.

Hildebrand, H. P. (1990). The other side of the wall: A psychoanalytic study of creativity in later life. In R. Nemiroff and C. Colarusso (Eds.), *New dimensions in adult development*, pp. 467–86. New York: Basic Books.

Horney, K. (1967). The dread of women. In H. Kelman (Ed.), *Feminine psychology*, pp. 133–46. New York: Norton. Original work published 1932.

Imber-Black, E., and J. Roberts. (1992). *Rituals for our times*. New York: HarperCollins.

Jacobowitz, J., and N. Newton. (1990). Time, context, and character: A life-span view of psychopathology during the second half of life. In R. Nemiroff and C. Colarusso (Eds.), *New dimensions in adult development*, pp. 306–29. New York: Basic Books.

Jaques, E. (1965). Death and the midlife crisis. *International Journal of Psychoanalysis* 46:502–14.

Jaques, E. (1981). The midlife crisis. In S. Greenspan and G. Pollock (Eds.), *The course of life* 3:1–23. Washington, DC: U.S. Department of Health and Human Services.

Jordan, J. (1990). Courage in connection: Conflict, compassion creativity. *Work in Progress*, No. 45. Wellesley, MA: Stone Center Working Paper Series.

Jordan, J. V., and J. L. Surrey. (1986). The self-in-relation: Empathy and the mother-daughter relationship. In T. Bernay and D. Cantor (Eds.), *The psychology of today's woman*, pp. 81–104. New York: The Analytic Press.

Jung, C. (1971). The stages of life. In J. Campbell (Ed.), *The portable Jung*, pp. 3–22. New York: Viking. Original work published 1931.

Kalinich, L. (1989). The biological clock. In J. Oldham and R. Liebert (Eds.), *The middle years: New psychoanalytic perspectives*, pp. 123–34. New Haven: Yale University Press.

Kelly, E. L. (1955). Consistency of the adult personality. *American Psychologist* 10: 659–81.

Kerns, V., and J. K. Brown (Eds.). (1992). *In her prime: A new view of middle-aged women*. 2nd ed. Urbana and Chicago: University of Illinois Press.

Koestler, A. (1964). *The act of creation*. New York: The Macmillan Company.

Kris, E. (1975). *Selected papers of Ernst Kris*. New Haven and London: Yale University Press.

Kubie, L. S. (1961). *Neurotic distortions of the creative process*. New York: Farrar, Straus and Giroux, The Noonday Press.

Labouvie-Vief, G. (1985). Intelligence and cognition. In J. Birren and K. W. Schaie (Eds.), *Handbook of the psychology of aging*, pp. 500–531. New York: Van Nostrand Reinhold.

Lebe, D. (1982). Individuation of women. *Psychoanalytic Review* 69:63–73.

Lerner, H. G. (1985). *The dance of anger*. New York: Harper & Row.

Levinson, D. (1978). *The seasons of a man's life*. New York: Alfred A. Knopf.

Lifton, R. J. (1979). *The broken connection: On death and the continuity of life*. New York: Simon & Schuster.

Light, P. C. (1988). *Baby boomers*. New York: Norton.

Lisle, L. (1980). *Portrait of an artist: A biography of Georgia O'Keeffe*. New York: Washington Square Press.

Livson, F. B. (1976). Patterns of personality development in middle-aged women: A longitudinal study. *International Journal of Aging and Human Development* 7(2):107–15.

Lowenthal, M. F., M. Thurnher, D. Chiriboga, and associates. (1975). *Four stages of life*. San Francisco: Jossey-Bass.

Ludwig, M. (1992a). Creative achievement and psychopathology: Comparison among professions. *American Journal of Psychotherapy* 46(3):330–56.

Ludwig, M. (1992b). Culture and creativity. *American Journal of Psychotherapy* 46(3):454–69.

MacPherson, M. (1985). *Long time passing: Vietnam and the haunted generation.* New York: Doubleday.

Mahler, M. S., F. Pine, and A. Bergmen. (1975). *The psychological birth of the human infant.* New York: Basic Books.

May, R. (1975). *The courage to create.* New York: Norton.

Meyers, H. (1989). The impact of teenaged children on parents. In J. Oldham and R. Liebert (Eds.), *The middle years: New psychoanalytic perspectives,* pp. 75–88. New Haven: Yale University Press.

Miller, A. (1981). *The drama of the gifted child.* New York: Basic Books.

Miller, J. B. (1976). *Toward a new psychology of women.* Boston: Beacon Press.

Miller, J. B. (1991). The construction of anger in men and women. In J. Jordan, A. Kaplan, J. Baker Miller, I. Stiver, and J. Surrey (Eds.), *Women's growth in connection: Writings from the Stone Center,* pp. 181–96. New York: Guilford Press.

Miller, J. B., and I. P. Stiver. (1991). A relational reframing of therapy. Work in Progress, No. 52. Wellesley, MA: Stone Center Working Paper Series.

Mitchell, V., and R. Helson. (1990). Women's prime of life: Is it the 50s? *Psychology of Women Quarterly* 14:451–70.

Modell, A. (1989). Object relations theory: Psychic aliveness in the middle years. In J. Oldham and R. Liebert (Eds.), *The middle years: New psychoanalytic perspectives,* pp. 17–26. New Haven: Yale University Press.

Moffat, M. J., and C. Painter (Eds.). (1974). *Revelations: Diaries of women.* New York: Random House.

Morse, J. (1978, Winter). Freeing women's creative potential. *The Gifted Child Quarterly* 22(4):459–67.

Murphy, M. (1992). Psychoanalytic treatment at midlife. *Psychoanalysis and Psychotherapy* 10(1):58–65.

National Advisory Mental Health Council. (1995, October). Basic behavioral science research for mental health: A national investment, emotion and motivation. Rockville, MD. *American Psychologist* 50(10):843.

Nelson, G. (1994). Emotional well-being of separated and married women: Long-term follow-up study. *American Journal of Orthopsychiatry* 64(1):150–60.

Neugarten, B. (1968a). Adult personality: Toward a psychology of the life cycle. In B. Neugarten (Ed.), *Middle age and aging,* pp. 137–47. Chicago: University of Chicago Press.

Neugarten, B. (1968b). The awareness of middle age. In B. Neugarten (Ed.), *Middle age and aging,* pp. 93–98. Chicago: University of Chicago Press.

Neugarten, B., and N. Datan. (1973). Sociological perspectives on the life cycle. In P. B. Baltes and K. W. Schaie (Eds.), *Life span developmental psychology: Personality and socialization,* pp. 53–67. New York: Academic Press.

Niederland, W. G. (1967). Clinical aspects of creativity. *American Imago* 24:6–34.

Noble, K. (1990). The female hero: A quest for healing and wholeness. *Women and Therapy* 9(4):3–18.

Noy, P. (1978). Insight and creativity. *Journal of the American Psychoanalytic Association* 26:717–48.

Noy, P. (1984–85). Originality and creativity. *Annual of Psychoanalysis* 12–13:421–48.

Nydegger, C. N., and L. S. Mitteness. (1991). Fathers and their adult sons and daughters. *Marriage and Family Review* 16:249–56.

Oates, J. C. (1975). *The fabulous beasts*. Baton Rouge: Louisiana State University Press.

Ochse, R. (1991). Why there were relatively few eminent women creators. *The Journal of Creative Behavior* 25(4):334–43.

Oldham, J. (1989). The third individuation: Middle-aged children and their parents. In J. Oldham and R. Liebert (Eds.), *The middle years: New psychoanalytic perspectives*, pp. 89–104. New Haven: Yale University Press.

Olesen, V. (1990). Self-assessment and change in one's profession: Notes on the phenomenology of aging among mid-life women. *Journal of Women and Aging* 2(4):69–79.

Orbuch, T., and L. Custer. (1995). The social context of married women's work and the impact on black and white husbands. *Journal of Marriage and the Family* 57:333–45.

Ornstein, P. (1989). Self-psychology: The fate of the nuclear self in the middle years. In J. Oldham and R. Liebert (Eds.), *The middle years: New psychoanalytic perspectives*, pp. 27–39. New Haven: Yale University Press.

Piercy, M. (1980). *The moon is always female*. New York: Knopf.

Piercy, M. (1985). *My mother's body*. New York: Knopf.

Piercy, M. (1978). *The twelve-spoked wheel flashing*. New York: Knopf.

Reinke, B. J. (1985). Psychosocial changes as a function of chronological age. *Human Development* 28:266–69.

Reis, P., and A. Stone. (Eds.). (1992). *The American woman 1992–1993: A status report*. New York: Norton.

Rich, A. (1981). *A wild patience has taken me this far: Poems 1978–1981*. New York: Norton.

Richards, R., D. Kinney, M. Benet, and A. Merzel. (1988). Assessing everyday creativity: Characteristics of the Lifetime Creativity Scales and validation with three large samples. *Journal of Personality and Social Psychology* 54(3):476–85.

Riviere, J. (1955). The unconscious phantasy of an inner world reflected in examples from literature. In M. Klein, P. Heinmann, and R. E. Money-Kyrle (Eds.), *New directions in psychoanalysis*, pp. 358–59. New York: Basic Books.

Roose, S., and H. Pardes. (1989). Biological considerations in the middle years. In J. Oldham and R. Liebert (Eds.), *The middle years: New psychoanalytic perspectives*, pp. 179–90. New Haven: Yale University Press.

Roosevelt, E. (1937). *This is my story*. New York: Harper and Brothers.

Roosevelt, E. (1958). *The autobiography of Eleanor Roosevelt*. New York: Harper & Brothers.

Rothenberg, A. (1990). *Creativity and madness: New findings and old stereotypes*. Baltimore: Johns Hopkins University Press.

Rothenberg, A. (1992). Form and structure and their function in psychotherapy. *American Journal of Psychotherapy* 46(3):357–82.

Russell, W. (1988). *Shirley Valentine and one for the road*. London: Methuen Drama.

Sachidanand, U. (1994, January 1–8). Gender question in modern Japanese literature. *Economic and Political Weekly*, pp. 35–37.

Sacks, K. B. (1992). New views of middle-aged women. In V. Kerns and J. K. Brown

(Eds.), *In her prime: New views of middle-aged women*, 2nd ed., pp. 1–6. Urbana and Chicago: University of Illinois Press.

Sarton, M. (1965). *Mrs. Stevens hears the mermaids singing.* New York: Norton.

Schaie, K. W. (1994). The course of adult intellectual development. *American Psychologist* 49(4):304–13.

Sears, P., and A. Barbee. (1977). Career and life satisfaction among Terman's gifted women. In J. Stanley, W. George, and C. Solano (Eds.), *The gifted and creative: Fifty-year perspective*, pp. 28–65. Baltimore: Johns Hopkins University Press.

Statistical abstract of the United States (1996).

Simonton, D. K. (1992). Gender and genius in Japan: Feminine eminence in masculine culture. *Sex Roles* 27 (3,4):101–19.

Steinem, G. (1992). *Revolution from within.* Boston: Little, Brown.

Stern, D. (1985). *The interpersonal world of the infant.* New York: Basic Books.

Stiver, I. (1991). Work inhibitions in women. In J. Jordan, A. Kaplan, J. Baker Miller, I. Stiver, and J. Surrey (Eds.), *Women's growth in connection: Writings from the Stone Center*, pp. 223–36. New York: Guilford Press.

Surrey, J. L. (1985). Self-in-relation: A theory of women's development. Work in Progress, No. 13. Wellesley, MA: Stone Center Working Paper Series.

Vaillant, G. (1985). Loss as a metaphor for attachment. *The American Journal of Psychoanalysis* 45(1):59–67.

Vaillant, G., and C. Vaillant. (1990). Determinants and consequences of creativity in a cohort of gifted women. *Psychology of Women Quarterly* 14:607–16.

Viederman, M. (1988). Personality change through life experience 111: Two creative types of response to object loss. In D. Dietrich and P. Shabad (Eds.), *The problem of loss and mourning: Psychoanalytic perspectives*, pp. 187–212. New York: International Universities Press.

Viederman, M. (1989). Middle life as a period of mutative change. In J. Oldham and R. Liebert (Eds.), *The middle years: New psychoanalytic perspectives*, pp. 224–39. New Haven: Yale University Press.

Wallace, D. B. (1985). Giftedness and the construction of a creative life. In F. D. Horowitz and M. O'Brien (Eds.), *The gifted and talented: Developmental perspectives*, pp. 361–84. Washington, DC: American Psychological Association.

Weenolsen, P. (1988). *Transcendence of loss over the life span.* New York: Hemisphere Publishing.

Weisberg, R. (1994). Genius and madness: A quasi-experimental test of the hypothesis that manic-depression increases creativity. *Psychological Science* 5(6):361–67.

Weisblatt, S. (1977). The creativity of Sylvia Plath's Ariel period: Toward origins and meanings. *The Annual of Psychoanalysis* 5:379–404.

Welsh, W., and A. Stewart. (1995). Relationships between women and their parents: Implications for midlife well-being. *Psychology and Aging* 10(2):181–90.

Williams, M. (1985). *The velveteen rabbit or how toys become real.* New York: Doubleday.

Wink, P. (1991). Self- and object-directedness in adult women. *Journal of Personality* 59:769–91.

Wink, P. (1992). Three types of narcissism in women from college to mid-life. *Journal of Personality* 60(1):7–30.

Wink, P., and R. Helson. (1993). Personality change in women and their partners. *Journal of Personality and Social Psychology* 65(3):597–605.

Woolf, V. (1929). *A room of one's own.* New York: Harcourt Brace Jovanovich.

York, K. L., and O. P. John. (1992). The four faces of Eve: A typological analysis of women's personality at midlife. *Journal of Personality and Social Psychology* 63(3):494–508.

INDEX

abandonment, 51, 134, 147, 148, 152, 169

Abzug, B., 68, 75, 89, 110

acceptance, 6, 18, 112, 121, 168, 175–176; of limits, 46, 194; of personal mortality, 36, 46; of responsibility, 38; of self, 113–115

achievement, 45, 68, 90, 122, 135, 140, 162, 191–194

Ackerman, R., 185, 188

adoption, 54–56

aggression, 64, 67, 125, 134–136, 140, 145–146; alcoholism, 6, 96; and creative living, 125, 136

Alice in Wonderland, 38

Andreasen, N., 68

anger, 7, 96, 105, 126–137, 155; and creative living, 9, 58, 64, 131; differs from aggression, 126, 134; during mourning, 17, 20, 130, 159; fear of, 145–146; and insurgency, 130, 136; as a result of subordinate status, 126; unacceptable in women, 127

anxiety, 50–51, 63, 68, 100, 102, 148–149, 180, 183, 194–196

Applegarth, A., 157

attitudes, 31, 37, 41, 100–101, 133, 150, 161, 178, 180, 185; changing, 57, 60, 173, 176; creative, 39, 45–50, 63, 65

Atwood, M., 191, 199

Auchincloss, E., 138, 200

authenticity, 44, 58, 65, 87, 97, 111–112, 121, 128–129, 136–137, 146, 152, 164, 175, 180, 193–194

Awakening, The, 85, 90

baby boomer, 7, 104, 109, 133

Baker, S. Josephine, 165–166, 169–170

balance of self and other, 44, 74, 84–85, 108, 122, 183

Baltes, P., 109

Barbee, A., 189

Barnett, R. C., 109

Barron, F., 72

Baruch, G. K., 109

Bateson, M. C., 105–106, 109

Baum, L. F., 170

Baumeister, R., 170

Begley, S., 68

Benet, M., 68

Berkeley Guidance Study, 138

Bernay, T., 89, 157

Black, S. M., 157

Block, J., 98

Breznitz, S., 138

Brown, J., 140

Bruch, C. B., 67

Cameron, J., 156, 157

Campbell, J., 47, 67, 109

Cangelosi, D., 68

Cantor, D., 89, 157

career, 34–35, 42, 75, 95, 129, 134, 166, 179, 184–187, 189, 194; balanced with family, 44, 88, 96, 102–103, 122, 194; early versus late start, 106–107, 135; paths, 71, 183, 185

Chafe, W. H., 101, 109

Chasseguet-Smirgel, J., 157

child bearing, end of, 37

children: and acceptance, 113; changing relationships with, 10, 12, 14–16, 19, 22–23, 41, 42–43, 74; as creations, 65, 97, 155, 191–192; and generativity, 45–47; leaving home, 33, 38, 67, 135, 139, 184; not having, 32, 107, 135, 161; problems with, 11, 153–154; protection of, 25, 118, 126–127; raising, 7–8, 72, 133, 135, 137, 174, 176; and working mothers, 181, 183

Chiriboga, D., 47, 139, 157
Chodorow, N., 74, 89, 90, 137, 157
Chopin, K., 85, 90
chronological age, 32, 47, 106–107, 109
civil rights, 99–100, 103
Clark, L., 47, 137, 141, 188, 189
Cohler, B., 123, 140
Colarusso, C., 123, 156, 200
confidence, 62, 81, 121, 129, 137, 168; increases in, 10, 12, 44, 75, 88, 133, 135, 139, 148, 150, 153, 172, 175, 180, 185, 192, 193; lack of, 88, 138–139, 169
connections: and creativity, 51, 52, 122; importance in women's lives, 74–75, 79; to others, 23, 74, 81, 86, 92, 165, 179, 187–188; to self, 83; to the past and future, 46, 95
conscious, 52, 71, 81, 83, 145; thought, 51, 161
Conway, J. K., 170
courage, 4–6, 115, 136, 172, 184; new definition of, 169–170; to relinquish illusions, 22–26; and risk-taking, 60, 162, 163–164, 194
creative (creativity): and anger, 125–126; attitude, 14, 39, 50, 59, 60, 133, 136, 170; and change, 14, 179, 183, 185–186; and healing, 155–156, 193–194; and immortality, 46; living, 112, 122, 177, 194–195, 199; and loss, 157, 197; and middle age, 143; and neurotic processes, 62; problems, 143–156; process of, 50, 63; professions, 63, 68, 198; thinking, 49–53, 58; women, 45, 61–66
Custer, L., 109

Datan, N., 109
death, 6, 9, 34, 38–39, 45–48; of child, 57; and creativity, 137, 157; denial of, 45–46; of parents, 55–56, 57
Dennis, W., 188
depression, 22, 33, 63–64, 68, 102, 137, 166
Dietrich, D., 157, 188

disabilities, 175
divorce, 6, 8, 22–23, 25–27, 85–87, 95, 102–104, 114, 116, 121, 128, 151; and anger, 130–132; promotes change, 169, 178, 195
dread of women, 84
dreams, 192–199; as guides, 97, 115, 159; last chance for, 184; Levinson's "adult dream," 194; of parents, 91, 95–97, 112, 147
Drebing, C., 199
drugs, 176; and artists, 63, 68; as an escape, 14

Easter Bunny, 167
Edelstein, L., 48, 89
empathy, 64, 65, 89, 122, 179; development of, 82
empty nest, 33, 38, 42, 62, 67, 149
entitlement, 7, 14, 112, 118–123
Erikson, E., 42, 44, 47
ethic of care, 75

failure, 45, 46, 120, 150, 155, 176, 178, 196, 199; examination of, 38–39; from lack of confidence, 169; imperfection as, 46; physical, 92
false self, 150
Feminine Mystique, The, 103, 109
feminist: contributions to psychology, 90; movement, 99, 103, 108, 166, 173
Fiske, M., 133, 138, 157
Frankel, V., 180
French, M., 109
Freud, S., 29, 84, 85, 89, 90, 181
Friedan, B., 103, 109

Galatzer-Levy, R., 123
generativity, 42–46, 191–193
George, W., 189
Gilligan, C., 74, 75, 89
Gilovich, T., 157
Goldberger, L., 138
Gooden, W., 199
Greenacre, P., 66, 89
Greenspan, S., 48, 199

grief, 46, 55–57, 103, 130, 157, 159
guilt, 9, 51, 92, 114, 121, 146, 155
Gutmann, D., 138, 140, 146, 157, 180

Heilbrun, C., 37, 144, 157
Heinmann, P., 89
Helson, R., 62, 67, 68, 123, 138, 139
Hildebrand, H., 200
Hill, C. E., 157
Horney, K., 84, 90
Horowitz, F., 188
Howell, J., 47
humor, 141, 174, 193; as sublimation, 64
illusions, 14, 23–25, 139, 157
immortality, 46, 137
individuation, 74, 78, 81, 82–84
insight, 10, 33, 50–57, 59, 68, 137, 171
integrity, 42–44, 97, 169–170, 192–194
intelligence: crystallized, 39–40; fluid, 37
interiority, 60
internalization, 76, 80
introspection, 51–52, 61

Jacobowitz, J., 143, 156
Jaques, E., 29, 47, 48, 199, 200
John, O., 68
Jordan, J. V., 89, 137, 170, 188
Jung, C., 31, 47, 59, 60, 66, 100, 109
justification, 102, 129

Kalinich, L., 48
Kaplan, A., 137, 188
Kelber, M., 68, 89, 110
Keller, H., 109
Kelly, E., 133, 138
Kennedy, F., 137, 187, 189
Kerns, V., 138, 140
Kinney, D., 68
Klein, M., 89
Koestler, A., 66
Kris, E., 66
Kubie, L., 66
Kutznik, A., 140

Leary, M., 170
Lebe, D., 90
Lerner, H. G., 130, 137, 138
Levinson, D., 32, 47, 162, 194, 199
Lieberman, M., 140
Liebert, R., 47, 48, 98, 138, 157, 200
Lifton, R., 44, 48
Light, P. C., 104, 109
Livson, F., 61, 66, 138
loneliness, fear of, 148, 149, 183
Lowenthal, M., 47, 139, 157
Ludwig, A., 68

MacPherson, M., 103, 109
Mahler, M., 89
Malony, H., 199
mastery, 64–65, 135, 139, 171; active, 140; passive, 140
May, R., 71, 72, 136, 141, 170, 180, 200
Medvec, V., 157
Merzel, A., 68
Meyers, H., 47
Michels, R., 200
midlife tasks, 33–47
Miller, A., 98
Miller, J. Baker, 90, 126–127, 129, 137, 188
Mills, J., 33, 47, 137
Mills College, 138–140
Mitchell, V., 47, 68–69, 138
Mitteness, L., 188
Moane, G., 67, 123, 138, 139
Modell, A., 157
Moffat, M. J., 188, 200
money, 183
Money-Kyrle, R. E., 89
Morse, J. A., 67
mortality, 13, 35–36, 44, 47, 195–196
Murphy, M., 47
mutual empowerment, 82, 164

narcissism, 121–122
Nelson, G., 90
Nemiroff, R., 89, 123, 156, 200
Neugarten, B., 47, 60, 66, 106, 109, 140, 188

Newton, N., 143, 156
Noy, P., 66
Nydegger, C. N., 188

Oakland Growth Study, 138
Oates, J. C., 72, 89, 156
O'Brien, M., 188
Oldham, J., 47, 48, 98, 138, 157, 200
Olesen, V., 188
Orbuch, T., 109

Painter, C., 188, 200
Pardes, H., 47
parents: aging and death, 38, 92–93, 107, 122; care of, 33, 62; relationship with, 18, 51, 65, 75–82, 93–95, 100, 132, 168; search for biological, 53–56; single, 103
personal boundaries, 83–84, 88, 194
Piercy, M., 85, 90, 98
Pollock, G., 48, 199
power, 65, 87, 105, 108, 136–137, 155–156
psychoanalysis, 51
psychopathology, 63
psychosis, 63, 68

reconnect: problems, 144, 149; to dreams, 13–14, 196–199; to self, 8, 71–72, 112, 171, 191
refocus, 186, 191; and interruptions, 32, 106; on the future, 6–7, 159, 163–164, 171, 194
regret, 164, 185; problems of, 150–152
Reinke, B., 47, 109
relationships: and anger, 127, 146; modification of, 40–42, 61, 74–75, 104, 132–133, 165; problems in, 85–88; unequal, 56, 80, 86, 101, 128, 152
restrictive thinking, 58–59
Rich, A., 16
Richards, R., 68
risk, 41, 186; and anger, 11–12; and creative change, 57–60; and time left, 150; and vulnerability, 116–118
Riviere, J., 79, 89

roles: changes in, 41–44; limitations in, 100, 104, 179, 195; multiple, 107–108
Roose, S., 47
Roosevelt, E., 94, 98, 172–175, 176, 180
Russell, W., 17, 29

Sarton, M., 109, 110, 181
Schaefer, C. E., 68
Schaie, K., 37, 47, 109
Schroeder, P., 188
Sears, P., 189
selfish, 75, 92, 118–121, 156, 187
Shabad, P., 157, 189
Shirley Valentine, 17, 20–21, 29, 175
Simonton, D., 68, 189
Solano, C., 189
solitude, 179
Stanley, J., 191
Stanton, E. C., 108
Stern, D., 89
Stewart, A., 98
Stiver, I., 90, 137, 182, 188
Stone Center, 89, 90, 137, 170, 188
success, 186–188, 192–198; definition of, 84, 102, 169; and failure, 27, 151, 176; and independence, 184; problems with, 155
Surrey, J., 89, 137, 188

therapy, 9, 51, 54–55, 80, 85, 105, 117, 143, 145, 147, 152, 154, 160–161, 168, 177
Thurnher, M., 47, 139, 157
time: historical, 106, 108; life, 106; social, 107
transitions, 62, 133; as bridges, 159–160; and insight, 50, 178; reflected in dreams, 106–161
Trosman, D., 89
turning points, 171–180

unconscious, 50, 55, 81, 145, 178

Vaillant, C., 48, 68
Vaillant, G., 48, 68, 90
Van de Kemp, H., 199

Velveteen Rabbit, The, 111, 123
Viederman, M., 138, 157, 188–189
Vietnam, 99, 103

Wallace, D., 188
Weisberg, R., 68
Weisblatt, S., 157
Welsh, W., 98
White, R. W., 72
Williams, M., 123

Wink, P., 62, 67, 123, 139–140
Wizard of Oz, The, 55, 163, 170
Women's Room, The, 105, 109
Woolf, V., 65–66, 68, 198, 200
work, 181–182; and creativity, 57–58,
    63, 71, 149, 197; patterns after
    World War II, 101–103; problems in,
    80, 155–156; and regret, 38

York, K., 67

About the Author

LINDA N. EDELSTEIN, Ph.D., is a writer and clinical psychologist in private practice in Illinois, and an Associate Professor at the Chicago School of Professional Psychology in Chicago. She lives in Evanston, Illinois and has two daughters. Dr. Edelstein would enjoy hearing from readers about their midlife experiences through e-mail at Midlifeart@aol.com.